Intermittent Fasting For Women Over 50

A Complete Guide for Beginners to Weight Loss, Living a Healthier Life, And a Younger Looking Self

ELENA WHEATLY

©Copyright 2021 by ELENA WHEATLY- All rights reserved.

This document is geared towards providing exact and reliable information in regards to the topic and issue covered. The publication is sold with the idea that the publisher is not required to render accounting, officially permitted, or otherwise, qualified services. If advice is necessary, legal or professional, a practiced individual in the profession should be ordered.

From a Declaration of Principles which was accepted and approved equally by a Committee of the American Bar Association and a Committee of Publishers and Associations.

In no way is it legal to reproduce, duplicate, or transmit any part of this document in either electronic means or printed format. Recording of this publication is strictly prohibited, and any storage of this document is not allowed unless with written permission from the publisher.

All rights reserved. The information provided herein is stated to be truthful and consistent. In terms of inattention or otherwise, any liability, by any usage or abuse of any policies, processes, or directions contained within is the solitary and utter responsibility of the recipient reader. Under no circumstances will any legal responsibility or blame be held against the publisher for reparation, damages, or monetary loss due to the information herein, either directly or indirectly.

Respective authors own all copyrights not held by the publisher.

The information herein is offered for informational purposes solely and is universal as such. The presentation of the information is without a contract or any guarantee assurance.

The trademarks used are without any consent, and the publication of the trademark is without permission or backing by the trademark owner. All trademarks and brands within this book are for clarifying purposes only and are owned by the owners themselves, not affiliated with this document.

Table of Contents

INTRODUCTION 7

CHAPTER 1: WHAT IS INTERMITTENT FASTING? 11

    1.1   How IF works? 13
    1.2   How much time will our body take to adjust? 15
    1.3   What does it do for the human body? 15
    1.4   Is IF different for women? 16
    1.5   Is intermittent fasting safe for women over 50? 17
    1.6   Why intermittent fasting? 18
    1.7   Who should not try intermittent fasting? 21

CHAPTER 2: METHODS OF INTERMITTENT FASTING 23

    2.1   16/8 23
    2.2   5:2 method 26
    2.3   Eat Stop Eat 29
    2.4   Alternate day fasting 32
    2.5   The Warrior Diet Method 35
    2.6   Spontaneous meal skipping method 38
    2.7   Lean gains method 40
    2.8   Crescendo Fasting 43

CHAPTER 3: BENEFITS OF INTERMITTENT FASTING 46

    3.1   Evidence-Based Benefits of Intermittent Fasting 46
        3.1.1   May Strengthens Musculoskeletal System 46
        3.1.2   It can help you lose weight and visceral fat 46
        3.1.3   Can reduce insulin resistance, lowering the risk for type 2 diabetes 48
        3.1.4   It can help the body minimize oxidative stress and inflammation 49
        3.1.5   It Might be beneficial for heart health 49
        3.1.6   Induces a variety of cellular repair processes 50
        3.1.7   It May help prevent cancer 50
        3.1.8   Intermittent fasting makes your day simpler 50
        3.1.9   Intermittent fasting is much easier than dieting 51
        3.1.10   Has benefits for your brain 53
        3.1.11   It May help prevent Alzheimer's disease 55
        3.1.12   May extend your lifespan, helping you live longer 56
    3.2   The Hour-by-Hour Benefits of Intermittent Fasting 57

CHAPTER 4: DRAWBACKS OF INTERMITTENT FASTING 60

    4.1   You are hungry 60
    4.2   Fatigue or fogging of the mind 61
    4.3   Obsessions with food 62

- 4.4 A low blood sugar level 63
- 4.5 Hair Loss 63
- 4.6 Constipation 63
- 4.7 Unhealthy eating habits 64
- 4.8 Sleep deprivation 64
- 4.9 Constant Changes in Mood 66
- 4.10 Lightheadedness and headaches 67
- 4.11 Problems with digestion 67
- 4.12 Bad Breathing 68
- 4.13 Dehydration 68
- 4.14 Malnutrition 69

CHAPTER 5: INTERMITTENT FASTING RULES 70

- 5.1 Begin gradually: Try Crescendo Fasting 70
- 5.2 Portion Sizes Should Be Restricted 70
- 5.3 Choose an Appropriate Eating Window 71
- 5.4 Experiment with a 12-hour feeding window 71
- 5.5 Eat Protein-Rich Foods 72
- 5.6 Drink Lots of Water 73
- 5.7 Do not Force Yourself to Workout Fasted 73
- 5.8 Keep Yourself Busy During Fast 74
- 5.9 Take BCAAs 74
- 5.10 Maintain Consistency 75

CHAPTER 6: TIPS AND TRICKS FOR INTERMITTENT FASTING 76

- 6.1 Tips to follow while Intermittent Fasting 76
  - 6.1.1 Eat Well During the Eating Window 76
  - 6.1.2 Add Fiber to Your Diet 76
  - 6.1.3 Crescendo Fasting is good for a start 76
  - 6.1.4 Check the hormone levels regularly 77
  - 6.1.5 Need to get in the Right Mindset 77
  - 6.1.6 Decide how you'd like to fast 79
  - 6.1.7 Maintain as much of a routine as possible 79
  - 6.1.8 Maintain hydration 80
  - 6.1.9 Maintain Portion Control 80
  - 6.1.10 Consume the Correct Foods 81
  - 6.1.11 Sleep Well 82
- 6.2 Weight Loss tips 83
  - 6.2.1 Obtain Enough Rest 83
  - 6.2.2 Strengthen the body 83
  - 6.2.3 Sugar consumption should be reduced 83
  - 6.2.4 Keep a food diary 83
  - 6.2.5 Take a probiotic supplement 83

CHAPTER 7: PSYCHOLOGICAL EFFECTS OF INTERMITTENT FASTING 85

- 7.1 IT HAS THE POTENTIAL TO AFFECT YOUR MOOD 85
- 7.2 IT MAY MAKE YOU FEEL EVEN MORE ANXIOUS 85
- 7.3 IT CAN MAKE YOU TIRED 86
- 7.4 IT CAN MAKE YOU LONELY 87
- 7.5 IT CAN INCREASE THE POSSIBILITY OF DEVELOPING EATING DISORDERS IN SOME PEOPLE. 87
- 7.6 IT CAN HAVE AN IMPACT ON YOUR COGNITIVE ABILITIES 89
- 7.7 YOUR PERCEPTION OF HUNGER MIGHT CHANGE 89

CHAPTER 8: REMEDIES FOR COPING UP WITH THE DRAWBACKS OF FASTING .. 91

- 8.1 HYPOGLYCEMIA 92
- 8.2 DEHYDRATION 92
- 8.3 ELECTROLYTE DEFICIENCY 93
- 8.4 CAFFEINE WITHDRAWAL 95

CHAPTER 9: MYTHS OF INTERMITTENT FASTING 97

- 9.1 MYTH 1: WHEN INTERMITTENT FASTING, YOU CAN'T FOCUS 97
- 9.2 MYTH 2: INTERMITTENT FASTING CAUSES THE METABOLISM TO DECREASE 97
- 9.3 MYTH 3: EVERYONE CAN USE IT 98
- 9.4 MYTH 4: WHEN INTERMITTENT FASTING, YOU SHOULD NOT DRINK WATER 99
- 9.5 MYTH 5: NO MATTER WHAT, YOU'LL LOSE WEIGHT 99
- 9.6 MYTH 6: INTERMITTENT FASTING WILL MAKE YOU INCREDIBLY SAFE AND FIT 100
- 9.7 MYTH 7: INTERMITTENT FASTING IS NOTHING MORE THAN STARVATION 101
- 9.8 MYTH 8: THE MOST SIGNIFICANT FOOD OF THE DAY WILL BE BREAKFAST 101
- 9.9 MYTH 9: INTERMITTENT FASTING CAUSES OVERREACTING 102
- 9.10 MYTH 10: IF YOU FAST, YOU WILL NOT GAIN MUSCLE 102
- 9.11 MYTH 11: LACK OF ENERGY IS CAUSED BY INTERMITTENT FASTING 103

CONCLUSION 104

Introduction

Extreme diets abound around the world. Dietary supplements were common in the 1990s. You were losing out on life's classic fitness boosts if you didn't get a juicer in the 2000s. Green tea pads that minimize belly have been sent to us. As a general, if anything is marketed as new and life-changing in the field of fat loss, it's probably just a gimmick to promote whatever is now popular. So if there is a trend to get behind, it's intermittent fasting. Throughout the last two decades, neuroscientists have been researching intermittent fasting. They believe that our systems have adapted to go without eating for hours or days. People used to hunt until they began to cultivate and then adapted to live and prosper for longer periods without feeding. They needed to hunt and gather fruits and berries, and it required a lot of effort.

It was really easy to keep a healthier weight in the past years. People started feeding, and they slept since no phones, and Television shows ended at noon. The portion sizes were much lower. More people were working and managed to play outside, getting more exercise in the process. Television, cell phones, video games and other forms of content are now available at every time. We stay up later to watch our favorite movies, play sports, and talk on the internet. We spend the whole time lying and snacking. Heart diseases, poor quality of life, diabetes, obesity and other diseases will be exacerbated by eating so many calories and doing too little. Intermittent fasting has been shown in scientific trials to change these phenomena further. It is a way of feeding, not a diet. It is a method of planning your meals so that you get the best bang for your buck.

Intermittent fasting does not alter your eating habits; rather, it alters the timing of your meals. When it comes to losing weight, women over 50 will have a difficult time. A variety of factors can cause this. The most common cause is a slowing metabolism. The higher your metabolism is, the more muscle mass you get. If performed correctly, intermittent fasting for women can be quite helpful. If calories are reduced so severely, hormones can become unbalanced. Women who want intermittent fasting must give heed to their diet's nutritional content. Or else, they risk losing the effects of IF and doing more damage to their bodies than health.

Post-menopausal are common in women in their 50s, and fat deposition in the waist rises. Belly fat is not only the most difficult to shed, but it is also linked to several health complications, including type 2 diabetes, elevated blood pressure, and heart disease. Intermittent fasting is an excellent way to stay fit and stable when avoiding those problems. Intermittent fasting has been shown in many trials to be particularly effective in lowering belly fat. This is due to a rise in the intake of growth hormone, which aids the body in fat burning. When blood sugar levels are down, HGH levels rise. If you pair intermittent fasting with adequate sleep and regular exercise, the resulting low insulin levels aid in HGH production and improve fat loss. When we age, we lose muscle mass and become less healthy than we once were. Intermittent fasting allows you to eat whatever you want. According to research, fasting has been shown to increase appetite and mental wellbeing and potentially deter certain cancers. It will also protect women over 50 from some muscle and joint disorders. The below are some of the general advantages that can encourage women over 50 to try intermittent fasting:

- Insulin sensitivity is improving in overweight women.
- Infection and oxidative stress are reduced.
- Ongoing weight reduction
- Increased lean body mass
- Stress response in the cells has improved.
- Increased nerve growth factor development improves cognitive function.
- Increased energy levels
- Loss of size and body fat
- Increased fat-burning ability.
- Reduced insulin and sugar levels in the blood
- Mental focus and concentration may increase

- Increased energy is a possibility
- Increased growth hormone is a possibility, at least for the short term.

Chapter 1: What is Intermittent Fasting?

Intermittent fasting has increased in popularity in recent years since many people find them simpler to stick to than conventional calorie restriction regimes. If you think about it, IF makes a lot of sense. Notably, since it takes relatively little behavior adjustment, intermittent fasting is one of the best methods for losing weight while maintaining a healthy weight. This is a positive thing as it means IF falls under the category of "easy at doing, but significant enough to make an impact." Enzymes in our gut start to break down we digest, which then become molecules in our bloodstream. Sugar and processed grains are easily destroyed into sugar, which our cells use as energy. If our bodies don't need it all, it's stored as fat. Sugar, on the other hand, can only reach our cells by insulin. Insulin transports sugar into fat cells and retains it there.

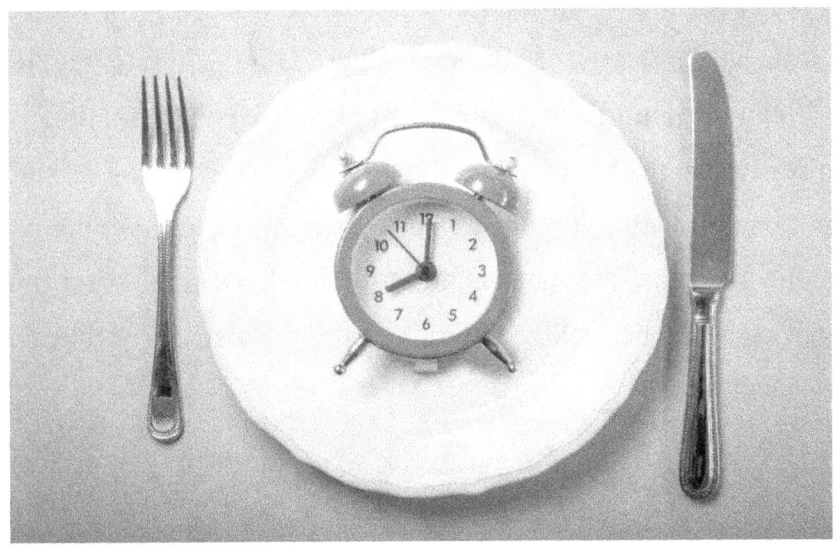

Our insulin level drops during meals if we don't eat, and our fat cells will release their accumulated sugar to be used. If we allow our insulin levels to drop, we lose weight. The whole point of IF is to cause insulin levels to drop low that fat is burned off. On restriction days, IF entails limiting caloric consumption for 3 - 5 days a week and eating openly on non-restriction days. Alternate day fasting is a form of intermittent fasting that involves switching between a "fast day" that includes 75% energy limitation and a "eat day" that includes an always available diet. Regular 16-hour fasts or fasting for 24 hours twice a week are two popular intermittent fasting practices. Fasting is much more natural than taking 3–4 meals a day. It is also practiced in Islam, Christianity, and Buddhism for spiritual or moral purposes.

Fasting is a method that can never be mistaken for a strict diet. There is also a lot to think about for women over 50 who want to resume intermittent fasting. When you decide to try it, gradually start and pay special attention to your appetite. If you're always hungry over the day or week, it's probably easier to get back towards a more normal eating routine. Keeping an eye out for signs like nausea, appetite, low energy. During the day, you should be fuelled, energized, and fulfilled, not lethargic and starving.

1.1 How IF works?

To comprehend how intermittent fasting contributes to weight loss, we must first comprehend the distinction between both the fed and fasted states. When the body digests and absorbs food, it is in a fed state. The fed condition usually begins when you keep feeding and lasts 3 to 5 hours as one's stomach digests and consume the food. Since your insulin levels are elevated while you're in the fed state, it's difficult for your system to burn calories. During that period, the body undergoes a condition known as the post-absorptive state, suggesting that it isn't consuming a meal. The post-absorptive condition continues until you reach the fasted state, which is 8–12 hours from your last meal. Since your insulin levels are poor, it is much simpler for your system to burn calories while you have fasted.

Whenever it comes to losing weight, there are two theories as to why IF might be successful. You may recall the popular "Biggest Loser" report, which was published in 2016. After six years, the study discovered that the volunteers had recovered most of their fat despite the previous remarkable weight loss. The metabolic rates also decreased, resulting in them burning even fewer calories than was anticipated. Another of the claimed advantages of this method is that it can avoid metabolic sputtering. Many individuals who want to reduce weight by diet and exercise fall off the wagon and gain weight. Hormones that stimulate excess weight, such as appetite hormones, are activated, and the theory is that intermittent fasting (IF) will help avoid this metabolic adaptation by tricking the system towards weight loss until it reaches steady. Fasting allows the system to burn fat that was previously unavailable during the fed state.

Our systems generate insulin to store glucose from carbs for future use as we feed. We exist in a world where most of our foods are routine, and we are forced to put up with foods that are rich in sugar and fat. This places anyone in an anabolic situation, which means we are still adding weight. Food glucose is processed as fat, resulting in obesity. Intermittent fasting effectively reverses this mechanism, allowing our bodies to use the glucose that has been processed in our bodies for energy. Fat loss occurs as cells reach a breakdown state. HGH (human growth hormone) is generated in reaction to the body's want for glucose, but when we eat often, our HGH output is reduced as we are receiving glucose from outside sources. HGH is a hormone that regulates metabolism and has many benefits for muscle regeneration and boosts metabolism. Fasting for short periods is said to increase HGH productivity by up to 5 times.

Our body systems are rarely in this fat-burning state, and we do not reach the fasted state till 12 hours from our last meal. This is why people who begin intermittent fasting lose weight without altering their diet, amount of food consumed, or workout frequency. Fasting induces a fat-burning process in your system that you seldom achieve on a regular feeding schedule.

1.2 How much time will our body take to adjust?

Intermittent fasting takes 2 to 4 weeks for the body to become familiar with it. When you are becoming used to the new schedule, you might crave sugar or irritable. However, researchers observed that when test subjects which make it past the transition process are more likely to adhere to the schedule and feel better. Water and zero-calorie drinks like black coffee and tea are allowed on days when you are not consuming "regularly eating" during your cycles do not imply "going insane." If you fill your meals with fast food, fried foods, and desserts, you are not losing weight or getting healthy.

1.3 What does it do for the human body?

Intermittent fasting does more than burning fat.

- Usually, prolonged fasting improves working memory and verbal memory.
- It can help with blood pressure, resting heartbeats, and other cardio metrics.

- A research was conducted where a group of people who fasted for 16 hours lost weight while retaining muscle mass.

- While in another research, it was found that overweight adult humans lost some weight by prolonged fasting in six small trials.

- Intermittent fasting is found to minimize tissue injury.

1.4 Is IF different for women?

Biological gender norms have influenced men and women's hormonal reactions to carbs, lack of sleep, and even fasting. Men and women reacted to times of abundance and shortage distinctly in hunter-gatherer cultures. Fasting resulted in a massive increase in metabolism in men, owing to their greater overall size. This metabolic increase provided them with the energy they needed to hunt. When men have not eaten much, their genetic code says, "Go find food for everybody. "According to research, human evolutionary adaptations to times of shortage can still be found today. Men's metabolisms improve by 14% during brief fasting cycles.

On the other hand, women do not react to intermittent fasting in the same way men do. Women's bodies reacted to times of shortage differently than male bodies in hunter-gatherer cultures. In surviving a long-term drought, women's metabolic rates slowed to save calories and store fat. What this suggests for today's women is that intermittent fasting might be the difference for them. Women are usually advised to fast for just 14–15 hours because they tend to do well with shorter fasts. Many women tend to be healthy by using modified forms of intermittent fasting. On the other hand, various studies have found that fasting days can cause hunger, mood fluctuations, loss of focus, decreased stamina, nausea, and bad breath. According to some reports on the internet, women's menstrual cycles have also been said to have ceased while on an intermittent fasting diet.

1.5 Is intermittent fasting safe for women over 50?

Females may benefit from intermittent fasting in particular. Since a female body has a greater percentage of fat than a man's, intermittent fasting seems to be an ideal option for women who are obese or want to lose weight more quickly. When striving to lose weight, the body will burn out food and starch reserves within about 8 -10 hours after feeding and only begins to burn fat for strength. Intermittent fasting could be the solution for women trying to shed weight despite maintaining a balanced diet and fitness schedule.

1.6 Why intermittent fasting?

We all fast or refrain from feeding for at least eight hours a day. It happens while we are sleeping. The conventional wisdom has long been that eating a hearty breakfast first thing in the morning is the best way to lose weight and improve overall health. However, new research indicates that taking a longer break could help with weight loss and improve your overall health. It is a growing phenomenon, but it is still evidence-based, with studies demonstrating its benefits. If you refer to it as "intermittent fasting" or "time-restricted diet," it entails taking a "break" from eating for somewhere between 12 and 16 hours per day.

For weight loss

It is a smart way to get healthy without being on a fad diet or severely restricting your carb intake. In reality, before you even start intermittent fasting, you will strive to maintain your calorie intake constant. Intermittent fasting is also a healthy way to achieve muscle strength when losing weight. The primary motivation for people to pursue intermittent fasting is to lose weight. Perhaps notably, since it takes relatively little behavioral adjustment, intermittent fasting is among the best methods researchers have for losing weight while maintaining a healthy weight. It is indeed a positive development as it implies that intermittent fasting fits the definition of "easy enough to do, but significant enough to make a difference." Early humans have practiced fasting.

When there was absolutely no food left, it was often done out of despair. When animals and humans are ill, they always respond quickly. Fasting is not "strange" because our bodies are perfectly capable of going without food for long periods. When you do not feed for some time, our systems go through various changes to help us survive during a drought. Hormones, genetics, and critical cellular repair pathways are all involved. When you fast, your blood glucose and insulin levels drop significantly, while your levels of human growth hormone skyrocket. People use so to increase their physiological wellbeing and will boost a variety of risk factors.

For living longer

Intermittent fasting has also been shown to help women live longer. It can prolong life as successfully as calorie reduction in rodents, according to research. It may also give protection against diseases such as type 2 diabetes, stroke, Alzheimer's disease, among others, according to some studies. Others like extended fasting because it is more convenient. It is a useful "new trick" that helps you simplify everyday life while still optimizing your fitness.

For flexibility

You shouldn't have to make food or prepare food for lunch when you wake up the fact, and you don't have to worry about food until 4 p.m. Intermittent fasting has another advantage to eat when you want. When 4 p.m. arrives, you don't have to think too much about what you're going to eat since intermittent fasting makes for a far more flexible diet. Even though you are on the road almost all of the time, you don't do any food preparation. It allows you to eat out and still preserve a photoshoot-ready physique. Intermittent fasting will suit you because it satisfies all of your requirements. It aids weight loss and fitness, combats jet lag, and is extremely convenient.

For Jet lag

Intermittent fasting, believe it or not, will aid in the reduction of jet lag. According to research, fasting for at minimum 16 hours helps remove what's known as our "food clock. "Dependent on light signals, our bodies operate on a 24-hour clock. This clock lets us know when it's time for sleep or eat, hence why we become drowsy in the dark and much more alert in the morning. If you move to a different time zone, your internal clock must adapt to the shift in signals, hence why you may feel exhausted and "off." However, the light was not the only signal used by your body to create these patterns. There are many other cues during the day that can help program your body clock, feeding. When you fast, your body's natural internal clock is reset because it doesn't have any eating signals to go on. If you then cue the body by eating simultaneously, you'd usually break your fast, but throughout the new destination body adjusts far quicker, and the jet lag symptoms fade away.

These are just a few benefits that why you should try intermittent fasting. A lot more benefits are discussed below.

1.7   Who should not try intermittent fasting?

Many individuals use intermittent fasting to lose fat, while others use it to treat medical conditions, including inflammatory bowel disease, elevated cholesterol etc. Intermittent fasting, on the other hand, is not for all. Before you try intermittent fasting or some other diet, make an appointment with your physician. Few people who should avoid experimenting with intermittent fasting:

- Those who have had an eating disorder in the past.
- Those who have diabetes
- Have some blood sugar issues.
- Are underweight.
- On medications.
- Have low blood pressure.

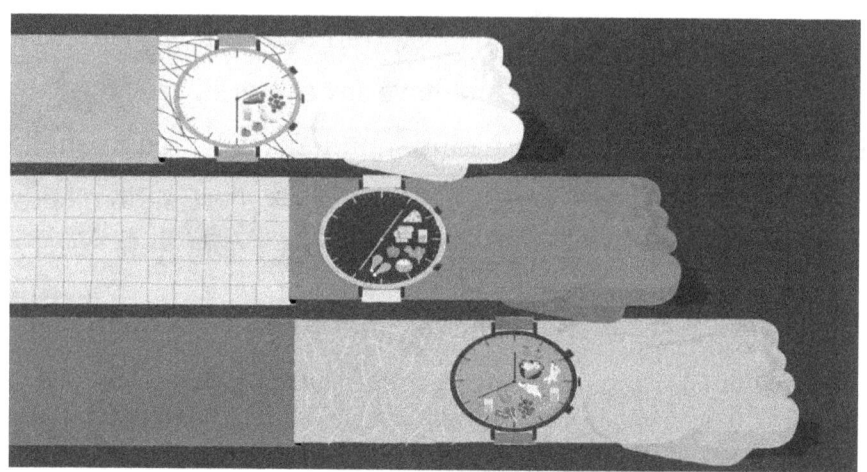

Individuals who are not in these groups and can easily go for intermittent fasting can go forever. It can become a lifestyle improvement with several advantages. Intermittent fasting can have various consequences depending on the individual, and it is not meant for everybody. If you have fatigue, discomfort, or other symptoms after beginning intermittent fasting, see your doctor.

Chapter 2: Methods of Intermittent Fasting

There are different types of IF to pick from. Choose the kind that best suits your lifestyle, and then discuss it with your doctor.

2.1 16/8

The method is used daily. This is the most often used IF form. A 16/8 is commonly used in the regular system. This entails consuming normal, nutritious meals for six to eight hours per day and then fasting for the next 16 to 18 hours. This has been discovered to be the most long-term form. You can eat 2-3 meals during the feeding time. Fitness gurus have popularized this form, which is also very easy to follow. It is as basic as not eating something after dinner and missing breakfast to follow this fasting process. If you have your last food at 8 p.m. but do not eat again until noon, you will have fasted for 16 hours. Others like to feed about 9 a.m. and 5 p.m., allowing plenty of time for a nutritious breakfast at 9 a.m., a regular lunch at midday, and a light evening meal or snack at 4 p.m. while you begin your fast.

You should experiment to find the Period that works best for you. It is important to focus on consuming nutritious foods during your eating window. If you eat a lot of fast food or consume an unhealthy amount of calories, this approach would not succeed. Try to provide a selection of nutritious whole grains in each meal, such as:

Fruits: Bananas, apples, berries, peaches, oranges, pears, and other fruits

Vegetables: Broccoli, cucumbers, cauliflower, leafy greens, onions, and other vegetables

Whole grain: Quinoa, rice, beans, barley, buckwheat, and other whole grains

Protein: Legumes, nuts, meat, eggs, poultry, fish, grains, and other sources of protein

However, when fasting, sugar drinks such as water, coffee, and unsweetened tea will greatly reduce your hunger while leaving you hydrated. Eating sweets or going overboard on sugary snacks, on either hand, may counteract the benefits of 16/8 and could end up causing more damage than good to overall health. It is easy to implement, adaptable, and long-term viable.

Pros:

Saves time and money: It is also useful because it will help you save time and money you spent cooking and food preparation. Not only does limiting your diet to several hours each day help you shed calories during the day, but tests indicate that fasting will also improve your appetite and promote weight loss.

Reduces insulin levels: It's been shown to decrease insulin levels by 34% and blood sugar levels 4–7%, effectively lowering the cholesterol levels. To get started, experiment with different timing options. A 12/12 diet involves feeding for 12 hours and then fasting for 12 hours.

Cons:

A problem in skipping breakfast: It helps reduce weight, but so many people out there cannot skip the first meal of the day.

Not enough calorie restriction: During the eight-hour cycle, you can eat quite enough calories and as many different types of food as you would like. This does not educate you regarding healthier eating and can lead to an increase in calorie consumption, which is unhealthy and can lead to weight gain.

THE 16/8 METHOD

	DAY 1	DAY 2	DAY 3	DAY 4	DAY 5	DAY 6	DAY 7
Midnight 4 AM 8 AM	FAST	FAST	FAST	FAST	FAST	FAST	FAST
12 PM	First meal	First meal	First meal	First meal	First meal	First meal	First meal
4 PM	Last meal by 8pm	Last meal by 8pm	Last meal by 8pm	Last meal by 8pm	Last meal by 8pm	Last meal by 8pm	Last meal by 8pm
8 PM Midnight	FAST	FAST	FAST	FAST	FAST	FAST	FAST

2.2 5:2 method

This method entails consuming regular, nutritious meals five days a week and restricting oneself to 500-600 calories two days a week. It's uncertain if eating all of your calories in one sitting or spreading them out over the day is better, so do what works for you. It is very easy to describe the 5:2 diet. You eat regularly for five days a week and do not have to worry about calorie restriction. You can cut your calorie consumption to a fifth of your normal requirements on the remaining two days. This equates to around 500 calories a day for women. One can fast every two days of each week you like. Fasting on Mondays and Thursdays with 2 or 3 balanced meals, then eating regularly for the remainder of the week, is a popular form of preparing the week. It is worth noting that eating "normally" does not imply that you can eat whatever you want.

If you eat fast food in excess, you will not lose weight and might even gain weight. You can eat as well as you would if you were not fasting at all. The 5:2 diet's versatility is a big part of its popularity. You won't have to obey any complex menu schedules, and you won't have to weigh servings or carb counting. To encourage fat loss and weight management, you can start consuming healthy foods on every eating schedule. To fill up your stomach on fasting days, continue to consume elevated, low-calorie foods. Carrots and broccoli, which are rich in nutrition, are excellent options for keeping your whole. You can drink whatever you want on normal eating days, but sticking to pure water or low-calorie drinks is the best option on fasting days.

You can try to stretch out the fasting days as far as possible. Eating a lot of high-volume foods can aid. If you are sticking to 500-calories a day, you might eat 200 calories for breakfast, 100 calories for lunch, and 200 calories for dinner. You might still consume 250 calories at brunch and only 250 calories at dinner. This is not easy to go from eating all day properly to just eating 500 calories twice a week. Begin by gradually lowering your calorie intake. Decrease the diet from 2,000 to 1,500 calories throughout the first week, for instance. Try just 1,000 calories the following week. Decrease your calorie consumption before you are taking the 500–600 calories needed on fasting days. If you have never experienced fasting previously, please remember that there's a fair risk you'll feel adverse effects on fasting days.

Pros:

Choose your fast days: You will feel more comfortable making healthier decisions if you concentrate on the timing of meals instead of the eating itself. You should select your fasts on the 5:2 diet, depending on your calendar. Most individuals fast during the week because it's easier to stick to a schedule, particularly if you've many social interactions on weekends.

No restriction of foods: Since no meals are legally banned, socializing with others can be simpler. It would also help you feel less hungry on days where you are not fasting.

Health benefits: It has been linked to various health impacts, including losing weight and better blood pressure and heart health.

Cons:

Difficult transition period: While the 5:2 diet can be manageable once you have gotten used to it, it does take some real commitment at first. In the first several fasts, you will probably experience extreme hunger and other side effects, including nausea and irritability. However, once you've gotten through the initial side effects, your body can adjust, and you'll feel more natural.

Overeating: Fasting often opens up the possibility of overeating. Not only can this lead to the negative side effects of binge eating, but it can also prevent you from achieving your fitness or losing weight.

THE 5:2 DIET						
DAY 1	DAY 2	DAY 3	DAY 4	DAY 5	DAY 6	DAY 7
Eats normally	Women: 500 calories Men: 600 calories	Eats normally	Eats normally	Women: 500 calories Men: 600 calories	Eats normally	Eats normally

2.3 Eat Stop Eat

This refers to a perfect 24-hour fast if you fast from dinner one day to dinner the very next day; for instance, you have done a perfect 24-hour fast if you end dinner at 7 p.m. Tuesday but do not eat again until dinner 7 p.m. Wednesday. The outcome is the same if you fast from dinner to dinner or breakfast to breakfast. During the short, liquids such as water and other low-calorie drinks are tolerated, but food items are not. You must diet properly during the feeding cycles while you are trying to lose weight. In other terms, you could eat as much as you would if you were not fasting at all. Since Eat Stop Eat is a form of intermittent fasting, it is designed to function in the same way as anyone else.

It will help you reduce your calorie consumption despite having you think about it too much. When you do not have as much time for lunch as you used to, it is much more difficult to consume the same number of calories in a week. Once you do eat, you will find it hard to overeat since your stomach has reduced slightly due to the fast. Eat Stop Eat can also help to kick start your metabolism. If you reduce the feeding time, you provide a fasting cycle during which the system must use its own accumulated glycogen from carbs and fats as food, and if those reserves are depleted, the body enters a ketosis and burns fat for energy. If you fast a long time, your body begins fat burning instead of carbohydrates for energy. Eat around 2,000 calories per day for women for the next few days; never fast on days in a row.

After a few days of regular eating, you can go on a fast again and continue the cycle. In any given week, do not fast more than twice. A calorie deficiency of 10% can be achieved by fasting even once a week. You are not required to eat any particular foods, such as carbohydrates; in reality, a limited diet on non-fasting days can reduce your energy. You should eat a variety of citrus, herbs, and spices. 20 to 30 grams of high-quality protein per 4 - 5 hours for a maximum of around 100 grams per day of protein. If required, any of which can be obtained from protein powder. If you notice yourself adding weight between fasts, reduce your food intake by 10% on non-fasting days.

Pros:

More muscle strength: The Eat Stop Eat method is almost as good at losing weight as reducing carbs by a certain percentage per day, and it also helps dieters keep more muscle strength.

Easy to follow: It might be less confusing and transparent than diets that need you to exclude a whole food category, such as fat or carbohydrates.

Cons:

Health issues: Few individuals may have headaches and irritability due to the diet, so it is not recommended for individuals with diabetes, pregnant mothers.

Increased cravings: Since you have "saved" calories, the package allows sugary beverages, making you want candy or prefer unhealthy foods.

There is no proper guidance: It makes no clear meal-plan guidelines for non-fasting days, allowing you to exercise incredible self-control and decide what and how to eat for yourself — an environment where many individuals are struggling with their weight need advice.

EAT-STOP-EAT						
DAY 1	DAY 2	DAY 3	DAY 4	DAY 5	DAY 6	DAY 7
Eats normally	24-hour fast	Eats normally	Eats normally	24-hour fast	Eats normally	Eats normally

2.4 Alternate day fasting

Often regarded as every-other-day dieting, switches four days of calorie counting (500 calories for women) with three days of eating openly. Consider it as a cycle of feast and fast so. For alternating-day fast, you shift between feeding and fasting days. Although experts are divided on the effectiveness of this solution to weight loss, the basic concept and promise of the method remain the same. Fasting flips the metabolism turn, so you start eating fat for food rather than the glucose contained in your liver. This promotes weight loss as well as other fitness advantages. Seeking an alternate-day fasting regimen that works for you can be difficult. Fortunately, there are a variety of alternate-day fasting schedules accessible.

On fast days, you can consume up to 500 calories and drink plenty of zero-calorie drinks as you want. To feel fuller for longer on fasting days, aim for 50 grams of protein and low-calorie vegetables like a salad with grilled chicken etc. You should eat anything you like and on feast days. It does not appear to affect what kind of food you eat as long as the overall calorie intake is limited. Many individuals do not overeat on feast days while fasting every other day. On feast days, individuals only consume 10% more carbohydrates than average, according to studies. Alternate-day fasters usually lose 5 to 10 pounds every three months, which is greater than most intermittent fasting methods like time-restricted eating, restricting eating times to a specific time a day.

On the ADF diet, when an individual loses weight, they burn fewer calories. This is not a symptom of hunger but rather a natural adaptation. According to one study, within six months of implementing an ADF schedule, people who are obese lose about 6.8% of their body mass. Intermittent fasting, on the other hand, may produce comparable weight loss effects as prolonged caloric restriction, according to a 2017 study.

Pros:

Autophagy: This form of fasting can also promote autophagy, a mechanism through which the cells eliminate protein build-up and dead or weakened cell structures.

Decrease in blood pressure: In this type of IF, studies have also shown reductions in **blood pressure** and **insulin resistance**, a precursor to type 2 diabetes that occurs when your body grows resistant to the effects of the hormone insulin.

Cons:

Time took: According to a 2017 survey, 15 percent of alternate-day fasters quit, compared with 26 % of daily dieters who limited carbohydrates. Not everybody enjoys calorie counting each day. It requires time to adapt to this feeding method, but in general, alternate-day fasters tend to gain hold of their appetite after about ten days.

ALTERNATE-DAY FASTING

DAY 1	DAY 2	DAY 3	DAY 4	DAY 5	DAY 6	DAY 7
Eats normally	24-hour fast OR Eat only a few hundred calories	Eats normally	24-hour fast OR Eat only a few hundred calories	Eats normally	24-hour fast OR Eat only a few hundred calories	Eats normally

2.5 The Warrior Diet Method

Among the first common diets to incorporate a method of intermittent fasting was the Warrior Diet. The Warrior Diet requires people to fast for 20 hours throughout the day and night, then overeat for 4 hours each night. This approach is founded on the assumption that our forefathers lived their lives by hunting during the day and feasted at night. During the fasting period, eat limited amounts of dairy, eggs, and raw vegetables to keep yourself going. Water, green tea are all zero-calorie or low-calorie drinks. To guarantee that you get sufficient basic vitamins and minerals, it is smart to eat a few portions of fruit and vegetables during the day. During the feeding time, there are no limits. Although you might order a burger, it is better to eat balanced, nutritional foods like fruits and vegetables. Throughout your feeding window, whole-grain foods, including sprouted wheat flour, quinoa, and oatmeal, are all excellent choices for refueling. Protein is recommended, and organic and full-fat dairy products; you can also have butter, yogurt, and raw milk.

Like in every diet, you can strive to limit a few foods and drinks, such as those rich in sugar and sodium. You can eat very little carbs over the 20-hour fasting cycle. Whenever it is time for your eating window, you can eat as much as you want before the four hours are up. You can choose your eating window based on whatever timeline fits best for you. However, most people prefer to eat in the evening. When it is time to eat, consider focusing your foods on healthy fats and significant amounts of protein, particularly milk protein sources like cheese and yogurt. The Warrior Diet eliminates the need for carb counting and thus emphasizes whole, unprocessed ingredients. Timing is a crucial aspect of this protocol. Long cycles of fasting and short hours of overeating lead to optimum wellbeing, nutrition, and body structure.

Since the Warrior Diet has no changes once you deviate from the 20:4, you are no longer on the Warrior Diet. There isn't much evidence to back up the effects of this form of fasting; intermittent fasting, in particular, has been related to a variety of beneficial effects, ranging from losing weight to increased brain health. While some individuals may benefit from the Warrior Diet, most will find the guidelines too complex to adhere to, but the Warrior Diet can be beneficial.

Pros:

May aid weight loss: As you fat for 20 hours, the ketosis will start after 12 hours and help you reduce weight regardless of whether you are eating anything for 4 hours.

May improve blood sugar: It helps in lowering your insulin that improves the blood sugar level.

May help with inflammation: Heart disease, asthma, certain tumors, bowel defects, and other diseases caused by inflammation. This form of intermittent fasting, according to research, can help combat chronic inflammation.

Cons:

Can lead to overeating: Fasting for 20 hours straight can result in extreme appetite and cravings, which can add to overeating and health issues.

Other health issues: Trying to deprive your body of significant calories will lead to nausea, difficulties concentrating, "hanger," mood fluctuations, depression, anxiety, lightheadedness, hormone disturbances, and other issues.

THE WARRIOR DIET

	DAY 1	DAY 2	DAY 3	DAY 4	DAY 5	DAY 6	DAY 7
Midnight							
4 AM	Eating only small amounts of vegetables and fruits	Eating only small amounts of vegetables and fruits	Eating only small amounts of vegetables and fruits	Eating only small amounts of vegetables and fruits	Eating only small amounts of vegetables and fruits	Eating only small amounts of vegetables and fruits	Eating only small amounts of vegetables and fruits
8 AM							
12 PM							
4 PM	Large meal	Large meal	Large meal	Large meal	Large meal	Large meal	Large meal
8 PM							
Midnight							

2.6 Spontaneous meal skipping method

You would not have to stick to a strict intermittent fasting schedule to enjoy any of the advantages. A further choice is to miss meals on occasion, including when you are not hungry or when you are very lazy to prepare and eat. It is a fallacy that people must feed every few hours or risk malnutrition or muscle loss. Your body is designed to withstand long stretches of hunger, much less missing 1 or 2 two meals now and then. As a result, if you are not hungry that day, miss breakfast and enjoy a nutritious lunch and dinner instead. Alternatively, if you are out and can't locate something you want to consume, go on a quick fast. A random spontaneous fast is when you skip either one or two meals when you seem like it.

During the other meals, make sure to eat nutritious snacks. If you wish to try intermittent fasting, remember that the consistency of your food is important. It's impossible to hope to lose weight and improve your fitness by bingeing on fast food at meal times. If you plan to start IF but do not want to leap straight in, meal-skipping is a good option. When you are not hungry, miss the meal next time. You may feel hungry, but it will pass quickly, particularly if you do not concentrate on it. To also have a good evening, work over the lunch break and finish an hour early. If you plan to skip a meal, avoid drinking something with fat content, such as juices or sodas. Instead, when fasting, sticking to low-calorie beverages like coffee, tea, and water is the best option.

Pros:

Flexible: it is one of the easiest types of intermittent fasting, and you do not need to go through the hassle of planning a meal.

Time-saving: you have to select a time for skipping a meal, and that's it.

Cons:

Slow weight loss: it is the easiest type of if, but unfortunately, you will see the results very slow. Usually, you will lose 0.26 pounds in a week and maybe 1 kg in a month.

Does not have a proper guideline: if you are trying to lose weight and are obese

SPONTANEOUS MEAL SKIPPING

DAY 1	DAY 2	DAY 3	DAY 4	DAY 5	DAY 6	DAY 7
Breakfast	Skipped Meal	Breakfast	Breakfast	Breakfast	Breakfast	Breakfast
Lunch	Lunch	Lunch	Lunch	Lunch	Lunch	Lunch
Dinner	Dinner	Dinner	Dinner	Skipped Meal	Dinner	Dinner

2.7 Lean gains method

A usual lean gains schedule begins with a one-hour exercise in the middle of the day. At 1 p.m., the exercise will be preceded by the start of the fed state. At 4 p.m., you will have your second meal, and at 9 p.m., you'll have your last meal. This lean gains ritual is famous since most individuals find fasting right after getting up to be easier. Fasting is made easier by the ability to take a cup of breakfast. A lean gains routine from 1 to 9 p.m. sounds like early morning and a late meal. Since it is a personal decision about which portions are larger or equivalent, it might be more prudent to have two larger meals and a smaller meal somewhere between. As a result, at 1 p.m., you would have enough strength to return from the fasting phase, and at 9 p.m., you should have enough energy to finish most of your activities for the fasting period.

It is essential to know that you don't have to follow this exact schedule. Everyone's routines and priorities are different. You can adjust the hours to fit your timetable as long as you're willing to fast for 16 hours. Regardless of the routine you choose, make sure to stick to it. The lean gains plan will be easier to adjust to if you keep a daily eating schedule. Black coffee, tea and sugar-free gum etc., are all acceptable within the fasting time because they have no calories. It is okay to apply a bit of milk to your cup, as well as something else that is still under ten calories.

The lean gains usually recommend a routine that replaces macros during the week. The carb and calorie consumption should be maximum on training days, with lesser carbohydrate and higher fat intake on non-training days. It is suggested that your post-workout meal be the biggest meal of the day. During rest periods, your initial meal might be the biggest of the day, responsible for about 40% of your total calorie intake.

Pros:

Flexibility: The simplicity that this method provides is a big explanation for many lean gains' successes. Any intermittent fasting plans call for only one or two big meals during the day. It is fine to be adaptable. Your progress will not be determined whether your initial meal serves 30 percent or 40 percent of your overall daily calories. If you like to eat the biggest meal at night and it reliably helps you achieve your goals, then continue doing what you're doing.

Improved metabolism: Responsive thermogenesis will cause your metabolism to slow down over the years. Short-term fasting, on the other hand, can potentially boost your metabolism. Fasting can also benefit your metabolic health by influencing signaling pathways that boost mitochondrial function, aid DNA repair, and enhance overall metabolic health. Ten. Fasting at night has also been shown to alter the gastrointestinal micro biota, leading to great metabolic health changes.

Health benefits: Intermittent fasting could combat disease mechanisms by triggering efficient cellular stressors signaling pathways Intermittent fasting has been shown to lower insulin levels by up to 32% and blood sugar levels by 4-6% in studies. As per a 2016 report, the lean gains procedure will result in better biomarkers such as lower insulin and blood glucose levels and lower body fat linked to higher energy consumption.

Cons:

Nutrition/Eating disorders: Prolonged fasting can be avoided by someone who suffers from an eating disorder. It is beneficial, but it may become a source of violence for those suffering from an eating disorder.

Stress issues: Individuals with a high propensity to stress must use caution before starting an intermittent fasting regimen.

Counting calories is time-consuming: Most people would not want to waste time measuring and calculating their food.

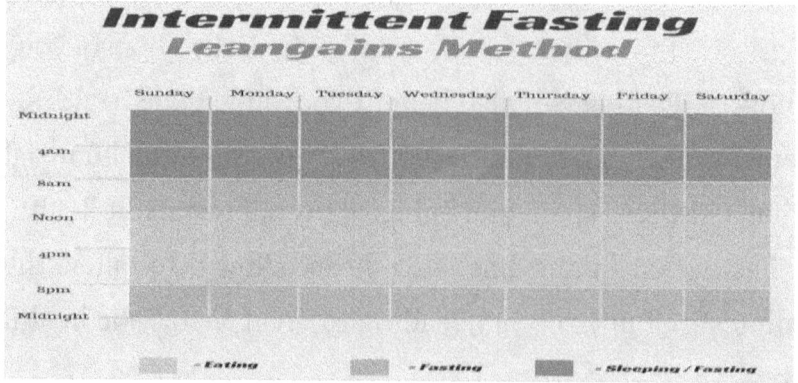

2.8 Crescendo Fasting

For women, this is one of the easiest and healthiest options. It is one of the most affordable methods for weight loss. It does not necessitate the use of additional instruments such as drugs, nor does it necessitate the use of pricey exercise facilities. What it asks is for strong and serious fasting self-control. The simple approach is to fast for 12 – 16 hours 2-3 times a week on alternating days. The "fasting window" 12-16 hours, and the "feeding window" is 8-12 hours. This method of fasting is a lot less difficult to adopt. Merely skipping breakfast is a simple way to get started.

You may encounter food cravings at first, but they will pass, and after you have become used to it, appetite will not be an issue. You will expand your fasting window to prolong the fat-burning Period during intermittent fasting while your system tries to adapt and your hormones stay healthy. You will probably understand that when fasting, you are concentrating, which is the exact reverse of what you would imagine, but it is something that most individuals feel. It is a gentler way of acclimating the body to fasting. When women fast in this manner, they can lose more weight while still gaining a lot of energy. Crescendo fasting can be performed twice a week on different days. This implies that you just fast 2 or 3 times a week. It is best to stop fasting on successive days. While you fast on Wednesday, for example, the next fasting days must be Friday and Sunday.

Drink lots of water during your fast to stay hydrated. One can also consume coffee, tea and a little bit of milk can be added.

Pros:

Reduces the risk of heart diseases: Intermittent fasting lowers blood sugar, lowers heart disease and stroke risk. In addition, crescendo fasting has been shown to increase blood pressure and reduces the risk factors for cardiac failure and multiple medical conditions.

Benefits brain: Fasting has been shown in several experiments to have profound effects on brain health. Fasting improves concentration and concentrating, response time, instant recall, intelligence, and the development of new neurons, among other neurologic advantages. Fasting has also been shown to decrease inflammation in the brain and aid regeneration post-stroke or brain damage.

Increases weight loss by accelerating metabolism: Often, calorie-restricted diets cause the metabolism to decelerate. Intermittent fasting, on the other hand, has the opposite effect. If we do not eat for a while, our systems will use surplus fat as a source of energy before we feed again. We start burning fat for energy, which promotes weight loss.

Decreases insulin production and the possibility of diabetes: Diabetes is prevalent, and its prevalence is increasing by the day. Diabetes is simply described as a disorder in which the system has an excessive amount of sugar. As a result, cells cannot respond to insulin and will not draw in more and more glucose from the bloodstream. Glucose levels rise as a result of these activities. It can help solve this problem in the system by reducing blood sugar levels, thus assisting in the reversal of insulin sensitivity.

Cons:

Might feel dizzy: Your body will take time to adapt to this routine, but while doing so, you might feel dizzy or feel strong cravings.

Can lead to overeating: Fasting for 20 hours straight can result in extreme appetite and cravings, which can add to overeating and health issues.

Chapter 3: Benefits of Intermittent Fasting

3.1 Evidence-Based Benefits of Intermittent Fasting

Here are ten evidence-based benefits of intermittent fasting.

3.1.1 May Strengthens Musculoskeletal System

Intermittent fasting has been scientifically proven to improve the general health of a skeletal system in women over 50. It has been discovered to be an effective method of reducing arthritis symptoms and back pain among older women. Changing meal plans as per intermittent fasting has also been shown to influence hormones that regulate bone and muscle health in a few studies. Fasting has been shown to help minimize pathways that increase the development of cancerous cells in studies. Intermittent fasting can help women over 50 boost their self-esteem and improve their moods while also reducing negative symptoms, including anxiety, depression, and stress.

3.1.2 It can help you lose weight and visceral fat

Many people who experiment with intermittent fasting do so to lose weight.

In general, intermittent fasting causes you to eat few meals. You will consume fewer calories unless you substitute by consuming even more during other meals.

Intermittent fasting also improves hormone function, which aids weight loss.

Low insulin levels, high HGH (human growth hormone) levels, and increased norepinephrine (noradrenaline) levels help the body break down fat and use it for energy. As a result, fasting boosts your metabolic rate, allowing you to eat even additional calories. In other words, it operates on both aspects of the calorie equation. It increases your calories expended (metabolic rate) while decreasing the food you consume (reduces calories).

According to an analysis, intermittent fasting can help with weight loss of 4 to 9% across 3 to 24 weeks. This is a massive amount.

Over 6 to 24 weeks, the study participants lost 4 to 7% of the waist circumference, indicating that they vanished a significant amount of visceral fat. It (Visceral fat) is the disease-causing fat found in an abdominal cavity. Intermittent fasting-induced muscle damage is less than constant calorie restriction, according to a 2011 study.

A randomized trial conducted in 2020 looked at the people who have used the 16/8 approach. You fast about 16 hours per day and the 8 hours to eat on this diet.

Fasting did not result in substantial weight loss compared to eating three meals per day. The researchers discovered that those who fasted lose a considerable amount in lean mass after checking a participant's section in person. Lean muscle was used in this.

More research into the effects of fasting on muscle loss is required. Overall, intermittent fasting does have the ability to be an effective weight-loss strategy.

3.1.3 Can reduce insulin resistance, lowering the risk for type 2 diabetes

Type 2 diabetes is on the growing more popular in the last few decades. The most noticeable symptom is a high blood sugar level, which is accompanied by insulin resistance. Low blood sugar can be improved by reducing insulin resistance and protecting against diabetic type 2. Intermittent fasting has also been shown to important benefits in terms of insulin resistance and blood sugar levels. In medical experimentation, fasting blood sugar in people with prediabetes was reduced by 3 to 7% over 8 to 12 weeks. Insulin levels in the fasting state have been reduced by 20 to 32%.

According to one study, intermittent fasting better survival rates and prevented diabetic retinopathy of mice with diabetes. Retinopathy is a disease that is linked to diabetes and can result in blindness. This means that people at the hazard of type 2 diabetes can find intermittent fasting extremely beneficial.

There might, however, be some distinctions between the sexes. Blood sugar control gradually deteriorated after just a twenty-two-day intermittent fasting period in a 2005 study of women.

3.1.4 It can help the body minimize oxidative stress and inflammation

One of the factors that contribute to aging and the development of many chronic diseases is oxidative stress.

It contains free radicals that are unstable molecules. Other essential molecules, including DNA and protein, are damaged by free radicals.

Intermittent fasting has been shown in many studies to improve the body's confrontation to oxidative stresses.

Intermittent fasting has also been shown in research to support fight inflammation, another major cause of many diseases.

3.1.5 It Might be beneficial for heart health

Heart diseases are still the world's leading cause of death. Various health indicators (also known as "risk factors") have been linked to increased or reduced risk of a heart attack. Intermittent fasting has shown to help with a variety of health issues, includes

- blood pressure levels
- cholesterol levels
- blood sugar levels
- markers of inflammation
- triglycerides in the blood

3.1.6 Induces a variety of cellular repair processes

If we fast, our bodies' cells start a process known as autophagy, a cellular "waste removal" process. Broken and damaged proteins that accumulate within cells over time are broken down and metabolized by the cells. Increased autophagy has been linked to reducing the risk of neurodegenerative and cancer disorders, including Alzheimer's disease.

3.1.7 It May help prevent cancer

Cancer is categorized by uncontrollable cell growth. Fasting is shown to have some metabolic benefits, including a lower risk of cancer. According to evidence from animal studies, intermittent fasting and diets which mimic fasting help prevent cancer. Human research has yielded similar results, but further research is required.

Fasting can also minimize the aftereffect of chemotherapy on humans, according to some evidence.

3.1.8 Intermittent fasting makes your day simpler

If you have been too hungry, you are well aware that an empty stomach can lead to irritability and rage. Spend enough time without food, thanks to intermittent fasting, and your mood will begin to change. Are you irritable? This is due to low blood sugar levels, "a spike of cortisol (the stress hormone)," which occurs when people are overly hungry. According to Ansari, blood sugar falls eventually spikes when "feasting"—can be particularly dangerous for people with diabetes because they can lead to a loss of blood glucose regulation and interfere with diabetes treatment and insulin requirements. (It is worth noting that low-carb diets such as the keto diet can benefit people with diabetes.)

Are you combative? That also appears to be right. "There seems to be a hormone named neuropeptide Y which causes people to be more aggressive when they're really hungry," Albers-Bowling says, "going back to caveman days when you just got to eat if you had been fighting or your dinner."

3.1.9 Intermittent fasting is much easier than dieting

Most diets fail not because we turn to the wrong foods but because we do not stick to the diet long enough. It is not a problem with nutrition; it is a problem with changing one's habits. That is where intermittent fasting (IF) shines because, once you get past the misconception that you will need to eat all the time, it's surprisingly simple to enforce. This research, for example, discovered how intermittent fasting was just an efficient weight-loss technique in obese adults, concluding that "subjects rapidly adapt" to the intermittent fasting regimen. The difference between trying a diet while trying intermittent fasting is the statement below from someone who has attempted intermittent fasting himself.

"Diets are easy to think about but difficult to follow. Intermittent fasting is the polar opposite: it is daunting to contemplate but simple to implement.

The majority of us have considered dieting. When we find the diet that appeals to all of us, following it would be easy. However, when we get down to the nitty-gritty, it becomes difficult. For example, I almost always eat a low-carbohydrate diet. However, if I consider going on a low-fat diet, it appears to be easy. Bagels, whole wheat bread and jam, corn, mashed potatoes, bananas even by dozen, and other foods come to mind, all of which sound delicious. However, if I were to start a low–fat diet, I would quickly become bored and wished I could eat meat and eggs. So, although contemplating a diet is easy, putting one into action over time is more difficult.

There is no question that intermittent fasting is difficult to contemplate. When we clarified what we were doing, people were surprised and asked, "You go without food over 24 hours?" "I'd never be able to do that." However, once you get started, it is a breeze. With one or two of the three foods a day, you won't have to worry about what to eat or when to eat it. It is a wonderful feeling of freedom. Your food costs drop dramatically, and you are not in the mood to eat. ... While it is difficult to conquer the fear of going without meals, nothing could be simpler once you get started."

3.1.10 Has benefits for your brain

What is beneficial for the health is frequently good for mental health. Intermittent fasting increases the number of metabolic characteristics that are linked to brain health.

Intermittent fasting aids in the reduction of intermittent fasting aids in the reduction of:

- oxidative stress,
- insulin resistance
- blood sugar levels
- inflammation,

Intermittent fasting has increased the production of nerve fibers in mice and rats, potentially improving brain function. Fasting also raises levels of a hormone in the brain named brain-derived neurotropic factors (BDNF). Depression, as well as other mental health problems, have been attributed to a lack of BDNF. Fasting has been shown to protect animals' brains from stroke-related harm. When you feed, some of the energy is stored in the liver. However, the glycogen levels would be extremely low but upon 10-24 h of not feeding. Consequently, you can become more agitated than normal, a condition known as "hangry." On the plus side, as your body's glycogen stores are depleted, fat cells throughout your body spill fats into the bloodstream. Fat cells are transported directly to your liver, in which they are transformed into energy for the body and brain. As a result, you're burning fat to stay alive. According to blood samples, people who fasted during 12-24 hours had a 60 percent rise in fat-derived energy, with the greatest difference happening after 18 hours. The advantage of intermittent fasting is that it places you in a condition known as ketosis. It's for this reason that scientists believe intermittent fasting may be the secret to living a longer, healthy lifestyle.

Ketones are chemicals produced as a result of fat burning. Ketones cause the release of BDNF, an essential molecule in the brain. BDNF aids in developing and strengthening neurons and neuronal connections in parts of the brain involved in learning and memory. This may explain why increasing ketone output has also been shown to enhance memory among people with dementia symptoms in as little as six weeks. For patients with serious epilepsy, growing ketones throughout the body is indeed a popular treatment. You don't have to quick to increase your ketone levels. Increasing your fatty food intake while reducing your carb intake may have a similar impact.

Several Women who used this procedure for three months lost weight and fat while lowering blood pressure and a hormone linked to aging and disease. However, scientists have found that fasting causes ketone levels to rise much higher. Ketogenic diets have also been shown to raise ketones 20 times, while fasting has also been shown to raise ketones four times. Consequently, fasting can have a greater, more beneficial impact on overall health than a ketogenic diet.

However, many Women eat food per day with snacks between in never hit ketosis and therefore don't produce enough ketones to be safe. From the beginning, fasting, as well as ketosis, have indeed been essential to our survival. They assisted our forefathers in surviving periods of famine.

They're now being known as a way to help future generations stay mentally and physically healthy.

3.1.11 It May help prevent Alzheimer's disease

The most severe neurodegenerative disease in the world is Alzheimer's disease.

Since there is currently no cure for Alzheimer's disease, stopping it from growing and spreading becomes crucial. Intermittent fasting has been shown in rats and mice to postpone Alzheimer's disease or reduce the severity. According to case studies, a lifestyle modification involving frequent fasts substantially boosts Alzheimer's symptoms for 8 out of 10 individuals. According to animal studies, fasting may also defend against neurodegenerative disorders, such as Parkinson's disease and Huntington's disease.

However, further human research is needed.

3.1.12 May extend your lifespan, helping you live longer

The most intriguing application for intermittent fasting is the potential to prolong life span. Intermittent fasting increases lifespan in rodents in the same way as constant calorie restriction does. Fruit flies have been shown to live longer when they fast intermittently. The results of certain studies were very dramatic. In a previous study, rats fasted every day now lived 83 percent greater than rats who didn't fast.

In a report, mice that did not eat every day saw a 13 percent improvement in their lifespan. Female mice's overall health was also improved by fasting daily. It aided in preventing hepatocellular carcinoma and liver disease, both of which are widespread in aged mice.

While it's far from becoming determined for Women, intermittent fasting is becoming very common in the anti-aging crowd. Given the benefits of intermittent fasting for various health indicators, it's easy to see how it could make you survive a happier and better life. Fasting boosts metabolism, allowing the body to break down nutrients as well as burn calories more efficiently. It also slows down DNA decay, which happens as we get older, and speeds up DNA repair, speeding down the aging process.

Fasting also raises antioxidant levels, which can help protect cells from becoming broken down through free-radical molecules that can cause cell damage. Fasting can also help to reduce chronic inflammation that develops as people age. "Intermittent fasting will help us live an improved way of life for a prolonged period," according to the researchers.

3.2 The Hour-by-Hour Benefits of Intermittent Fasting

Here is how your body works during an hour's fasting (times are dependent on your last calorie intake):

4 to 8 hours

Blood sugar levels drop.

The stomach is empty of all food.

Insulin is not made anymore.

12 hrs.

The food that was eaten was charred.

The digestive system is dozing off.

The body starts the healing process.

Human Growth Hormone (HGH) levels start to rise.

To keep blood sugar levels in check, glucagon is released.

14-hour time limit

The body has switched to burning stored fat for energy.

Human Growth Hormone (HGH) levels begin to rise dramatically.

16-hour Period

The body begins to increase fat burning.

18-hour Period

Human Growth Hormone levels begin to rise.

24-hours Period

The process of autophagy begins.

Both glycogen stocks are depleted.

Ketones are a form of ketone that is released into the bloodstream.

36-hour time limit

Autophagy has increased by 300 percent.

48-hour time limit

The rate of autophagy increases by 30%.

Reset and regeneration of the immune system

Inflammation response is reduced to a greater extent.

72-hour time limit

Autophagy reaches its limit.

* Autophagy is a detoxification mechanism in which the body removes damaged cells and regenerates new ones. Autophagy is

induced when a peptide p62 is activated, and it is a good way to increase life span over time.

You could fast for as long as you want, so you can do it every day or just once or twice a week or once a fortnight – the health benefits would be proportional to what you're doing and how much you do it.

Chapter 4: Drawbacks of intermittent fasting

As previously stated, the benefits of intermittent fasting are being studied, but there are some positive results. However, there is more than enough anecdotal evidence that intermittent fasting has some potentially harmful side effects, and you must discuss them with your doctor before embarking on an intermittent fasting eating plan.

Here are ten red flags to be aware of. If you experience any of the other side effects, you should immediately pause intermittent fasting and consult with your doctor or even a nutritionist before continuing.

4.1 You are hungry

We're not sure if "hungriness" is a real term, but it is undoubtedly a real sensation. This is the grumpiness, irritability, or general irritability from not eating while your body indicates that you are hungry. Training the body to go Sixteen hours without food requires some practice, and some people's bodies can never be satisfied with eating within such a narrow window. In principle, you shouldn't be hungry first thing every morning if you eat enough protein later during the day or night. If you are, that's a sign that you need to undergo some dietary changes during your calorie intake cycle to stop being a total jerk—or that's a sign that fasting isn't working for you. Not eating for long periods might not be suitable for certain people (e.g., those who work out a lot), which is worth considering. Don't try to push it.

You can feel increased hunger if you minimize your calorie consumption or go long stretches without eating. Some 112 people were randomly allocated to either an intermittent energy limitation category in a survey. For a year, they ate 400 and perhaps 600 calories on two non-consecutive days per week. These individuals reported feeling more hungry than those who followed a low-calorie diet with constant calorie restriction. According to studies, hunger is a common symptom people encounter within the first few days of such a fasting regimen.

In a 2020 survey, 1,422 people took part in fasting regimens that lasted 4–21 days. Only in the first several days of the regimens did they experience hunger symptoms. As a result, hunger symptoms can fade as your body adjusts to normal fasting periods.

4.2 Fatigue or fogging of the mind

Have you ever woken up in the middle of the morning, yawning uncontrollably, only to realize you'd forgotten to eat breakfast? Most people do intermittent fasting by skipping breakfast, noticing that you're always tired or making mistakes because of brain fog is a sign that you're not consuming the right foods throughout non-fasting hours. Fasting isn't working for you. You should pay more attention to what you're putting into your body. On intermittent fasting, you can eat whatever you want, but you really should still fuel it with nutritious foods that make you feel safe and strong. Listen to your body if you simply feel *much* healthier eating breakfast most days.

Intermittent fasting can make you feel exhausted and weak due to low blood sugar. In addition, intermittent fasting can cause sleep disturbances in some people, resulting in fatigue during the day. On the other hand, intermittent fasting has been shown in some studies to reduce fatigue, particularly as your body adapts to daily fasting periods.

4.3 Obsessions with food

Being on a restricted diet may affect your relationship with food. While some people enjoy the strictness of intermittent fasting, others can find themselves obsessing about what they should eat and how many calories should consume. Spending too much time worrying about the quality and quantity of the food daily can lead to orthorexia, an eating disorder. As per the National Eating Disorders Association, orthorexia is a condition where you place such a high value on "right" or "healthy" eating to hurt your overall health. The aim of any diet should be to form a safe, meaningful relationship with food, not to lose weight.

4.4 A low blood sugar level

Suppose you experience constant nausea, headache, or dizziness while on the intermittent fasting diet; it's a red flag that your blood sugar is out of whack. People with diabetes may avoid any form of a fasting diet for this purpose, as previously stated by WH: Hypoglycemia, a risky condition for those with insulin and otherwise thyroid issues, may be caused by intermittent fasting.

4.5 Hair Loss

Is this for real? Yes. Hair loss can be caused by unexpected weight loss or even an absence of appropriate nutrients, particularly protein and B vitamins. Although intermittent fasting (IF) does not always result in nutritional loss, it is more difficult to eat a well-balanced diet when you are cramming a full day's worth of eating into a few hours. Re-evaluate the nutrient quality of the daily meals and consult with the doctor about whether this is a good decision for you if you notice more hair falling out from the shower than normal.

4.6 Constipation

Is it all backed up? It's possible that intermittent fasting is to blame. "If you don't get enough fluid, vitamins, proteins, or fiber, any deficiency can reduce an upset stomach. People sometimes recommend drinking water during fasting hours, but going 16 hours without enough fluid would be a recipe for (gastrointestinal) disaster. So, if you've begun an intermittent fasting diet and aren't having normal bowel movements, it's time to put your plan on hold and talk to a nutritionist or doctor about what's going on.

4.7 Unhealthy eating habits

Even if IF (intermittent fasting) does not cause a severe illness such as orthorexia, it may also lead to poor eating behaviors. You also can find yourself making poor nutritional decisions during non-fasting hours, in addition to not having enough nutrients. "The biggest concern is that you'll start binge-eating because you're so hungry," Charlie Seltzer. If this describes you, you may benefit from working with such an RD to develop a plan that doesn't require you to limit your eating hours instead and focuses on providing your body with the nutrients it needs every day, not just at those hours.

4.8 Sleep deprivation

According to some studies, sleep disturbances, including an inability to fall or remain asleep, are among the common side effects of intermittent fasting. In a 2020 survey, 1,422 people took part in fasting regimens that lasted 4–21 days. Fasting caused sleep disturbances in 15% of the participants, according to the report. This was mentioned more often than other side effects. Since your body excretes large quantities of water and salt through the urine, fatigue can be more normal in the early days of even an intermittent fasting regimen. Dehydration, as well as low salt levels, can result as a result of this.

Other studies, on the other hand, have found that intermittent fasting has little effect on sleep. Research published in 2021 looked at 31 obese people who fasted on alternating days while still eating a low-carb diet over six months. According to the report, this routine did not affect sleep quality and duration or insomnia severity. Similar findings were found in a study conducted in 2021.

Many people report better sleep patterns when doing IF, probably because IF allows curbing late-night snacking behaviors, leading to an inability to drift off to sleep because the stomach is still digesting the 10 p.m. snack. However, some evidence suggests that the opposite is true. Evidence suggests that circadian rhythms intermittent fasting (daytime fasting) reduces rapid-eye-movement (REM) sleep, according to a study published in the journal Science and Nature of Sleep in 2018. According to the Harvard Business Review, getting sufficient REM sleep has been related to various health effects, including improved memory, cognition, and attention. It's unclear why this is the case.

If you're having trouble falling or staying asleep after starting an IF (intermittent fasting) balanced diet, pause and consult a professional to ensure you're not harming your health.

4.9 Constant Changes in Mood

It'd be odd if you didn't have mood swings or hungriness throughout intermittent fasting, at least at first. Although some people experience a significant increase in energy or motivation after adjusting to fasting, it's important to keep in mind that it's still a restricted diet. Feeling obliged to stick to it might make you depressed, particularly if you're isolating yourself from friends or family due to your dietary restrictions. Stop and speak with a licensed dietitian, counselor, or wellness coach right away if you're feeling down, nervous, or discouraged about intermittent fasting. They might assist you in developing a fasting regimen that is more suitable for your body and mind.

When people practice intermittent fasting, they can experience irritability as well as other mood swings. When the blood sugar levels are poor, you can become irritable. Hypoglycemia, or low blood sugar, can occur throughout periods with calorie restriction or fasting. Irritability, anxiety, and low focus are all possible outcomes. A 2016 study of 52 women was found during an eighteen-hour fasting cycle, and participants were substantially more irritable than after a non-fasting period. Interestingly, the researchers discovered that, while the women were irritable at the end of the fasting era, they also felt a greater sense of accomplishment, dignity, and self-control than they did initially.

4.10 Lightheadedness and headaches

Intermittent fasting is also linked with headaches. They usually happen in those last few days or even a fasting regimen. In a study published in 2020, researchers looked through 18 studies involving people who practiced intermittent fasting. Any participants in the four studies who reported side effects said they had moderate headaches.

Researchers also discovered that "fasting headaches" are normally located throughout the brain's frontal area, with mild to moderate pain in severity.

Furthermore, people who suffer from headaches are often more likely to suffer from headaches when fasting than those that do not. According to research, low blood sugar and caffeine withdrawal can lead to headaches throughout intermittent fasting.

4.11 Problems with digestion

If you are doing intermittent fasting, you can experience digestive problems such as constipation, diarrhea, nausea, and bloating. The reduction of food intake that certain intermittent fasting regimens entail can have a detrimental impact on your digestion, resulting in constipation and other unpleasant side effects. Additionally, dietary changes associated with intermittent fasting programs can result in bloating and diarrhea. Constipation may be exacerbated by dehydration, another popular side effect of intermittent fasting. As a result, it is important to remain well hydrated while fasting intermittently. Constipation can be avoided by eating nutrient-dense, fiber-rich foods.

4.12 Bad Breathing

Bad breath is also an unwanted side effect that some people experience when they fast intermittently. Lack salivary flow and an increase in acetone throughout the breath trigger this. Fasting allows the body to burn fat as a source of energy. Since acetone would be a by-product of fat metabolism, it rises in the blood and breath when you fast.

Dehydration, a sign of intermittent fasting, may also trigger a dry mouth, leading to bad breath.

4.13 Dehydration

As previously mentioned, the body releases a lot of water and salt in the urine during the first few days of fasting. Natural diuresis, also known as fasting natriuretic, is the name given to this operation. You might become dehydrated if something happens with you and you do not restore the fluids and electrolytes lost by urine. In addition, people who practice intermittent fasting can fail to drink or drink insufficiently. This is particularly true when you first start an intermittent fasting program. Drink water during the day and keep an eye on the color of your urine to stay properly hydrated. It should ideally be the color of pale lemonade. You could be dehydrated if your urine is dark in color.

4.14 Malnutrition

Intermittent fasting, if performed incorrectly, will result in malnutrition. Malnutrition can occur when an individual fast for long periods and does not replenish the body with enough nutrients. The same can be said for unplanned, long-term energy restriction diets. On different forms of intermittent fasting systems, people can usually fulfill their calorie and nutrient requirements. However, suppose you do not properly schedule or execute the fasting regimen for a long time or intentionally limit calories to an excessive amount. In that case, you risk malnutrition and other health problems. That is why, when fasting intermittently, it is important to eat a well-balanced, healthy diet. Make sure you are not restricting your calorie consumption too much.

A healthcare professional familiar with intermittent fasting will assist you in developing a health plan that offers the right number of calories and nutrients for you.

Chapter 5: Intermittent Fasting Rules

Follow these ten guidelines to ensure you are on the right track, whether you're new to intermittent fasting and if you've been doing it for a while and it's not working out for you.

5.1   Begin gradually: Try Crescendo Fasting

Crescendo fasting entails only fasting several days a week rather than every day. You will gradually introduce the body to fasting this way, ensuring that you stay committed to it.

The commonly used method would be to fast over 12 – 16 hours twice or three times a week on alternating days. The "fasting window" for this form of fasting is 12-16 hours, and the "feeding window" is 8-12 hours. This method of fasting is a lot less difficult to adopt. Simply skipping breakfast is a simple way to get started.

When fasting becomes approached in this manner, you will lose more weight while still gaining a lot of energy. In addition, crescendo fasting becomes safer, more natural, and puts the body under less stress.

5.2   Portion Sizes Should Be Restricted

What would you do if you have already limited your meals to 12 hours per day but aren't seeing any results? Consider limiting the amount of food you eat. To see the full benefits of intermittent fasting, most experts recommend limiting the daily food consumption to two meals a day.

This rule is especially important for people who are overweight or obese since they tend to overeat whenever they break or finish their fast. So, if you want to lose weight quickly, pay attention to your portion sizes and begin calorie restriction.

5.3 Choose an Appropriate Eating Window

Keep in mind that everyone's needs and routines are different, and there is no one-size-fits-all eating window. People who exercise every morning tend to go to bed hungry, while others cannot sleep without a proper meal.

So, rather than blindly following others, try creating your schedule. If you prefer to eat dinner with your mates, you can shift your mealtime from 12 to 8 p.m. However, if you cannot start a day with no breakfast, this same eating window could be from 8 a.m. to 4 p.m.

Do whatever works the best for you, as well as follow it religiously.

5.4 Experiment with a 12-hour feeding window

Although some people say that a 24-hour fast is ideal for them, expert's advice against taking such a drastic approach. It is usually recommended to refrain from fasting for longer periods on an even regular basis.

What is the reason for this?

According to the experts, limiting your food intake for six hours regularly may raise the risk for gallstone formation. This raises the risk of complications, including the need for gallbladder removal.

Fasting for extended periods has also been shown in studies to raise the risk for gallstone development in women, regardless of their weight.

Maintaining a 12-hour feeding window (no or less 8 hours) is usually considered healthy and can result in successful fat loss.

5.5 Eat Protein-Rich Foods

Alternate-day fasting has several negative consequences, including a significant impact on the body muscles, leading to muscle wasting. To compensate, increase the amount of protein throughout your meals.

Protein-rich meals may not only help you retain muscle mass, but they can also help you curb your appetite. Good foods to be included in your daily meals include chicken, eggs, oats, as well as nuts.

5.6 Drink Lots of Water

It is important to remember to drink water during the day. During your fasting period, please ensure you drink plenty of water. This is especially significant for people who have only recently begun to practice intermittent fasting.

You should drink black coffee, unsweetened tea in addition to water. Milk and sweeteners should not be added to your drinks because they can break your fast.

5.7 Do not Force Yourself to Workout Fasted

Many people enjoy fasted workouts. In a fasted state, they feel more energized and like they can devote more time to their training sessions. This, however, may not be what that everybody can do. Some people like to change their eating window so that they can eat before exercising. This is completely acceptable.

Whatever you choose, keep in mind that you can only exercise when you are at ease. This is necessary to ensure which you complete the workout session safely.

It is important to remember which fasted workouts aren't needed to reap the benefits of intermittent fasting. This is optional, and it is up to you to determine whether or not you want to do it.

5.8   Keep Yourself Busy During Fast

It is common to feel weird not eating when you are starting on an intermittent fasting journey. Long-term dietary habits and routines are primarily to blame. You might notice that you eat out of habit rather than need most of the time.

So, to avoid succumbing to the unwanted temptations by eating and out habit on fasting days, continue to put yourself occupied. If you do not have a job, consider picking up a hobby and keep your mind busy. To take your mind off food, read a book, call a friend, or go for a walk outside.

5.9   Take BCAAs

Intermittent fasting will cause muscle loss if you fast for long periods and miss meals. Taking BCAAs has been the only step to prevent this problem.

BCAAs (branched-chain amino acids) can be highly beneficial to people who fast intermittently. These proteins penetrate your bloodstream and aid in the development of muscle tissue.

Furthermore, BCAAs get the ability to circumvent the liver's degradation process and penetrate the bloodstream directly. As a result, they can be a perfect way to get instant energy without consuming something.

5.10 Maintain Consistency

It is not easy to begin an intermittent fasting diet. When your body adjusts to fasting, you may feel dizzy, fatigued with low blood sugar, or have other minor issues. Although these symptoms usually subside after the first week of fasting, they may be difficult to deal with. During the fasting window, you may notice yourselves slipping up and feeding. But keep in mind that it is all right.

All you have to do now is remain consistent, and you'll be fine. It requires time for the body to adjust to intermittent fasting, so make mistakes until then. Keeping a journal is one way to keep on track.

Chapter 6: Tips and Tricks For Intermittent Fasting

6.1 Tips to follow while Intermittent Fasting

6.1.1 Eat Well During the Eating Window

It has been said that everyone can fast, but still, it takes intelligence to crack it. After breaking a fast, what an individual eats is extremely important. A large green salad bowl with raw vegetables dipped in olive oil and steamed broccoli, spinach, or baked yam will be the ideal breakfast meal. Vegetables are commonly favored because they are low in calories and high in nutrients. Often, aim to consume a nutritious diet with a variety of nutrients during the eating window.

6.1.2 Add Fiber to Your Diet

Women over 50 may find intermittent fasting difficult, particularly if they have not encountered hunger for several hours per day. During the eating window, eating foods high in fiber and protein may help combat this issue. Fiber makes you feel complete and will help you avoid a blood sugar drop. Pasta, whole-grain bread, nuts, as well as beans are also good sources of fiber.

6.1.3 Crescendo Fasting is good for a start

Beginner fasters should begin with the crescendo approach because it establishes more manageable objectives. It is the preferred method of fasting for women because it ensures that hormone levels do not fluctuate excessively. This technique ensures that beginners get the most from intermittent fasting because it is a much gentler way to intermittent fasting.

6.1.4   Check the hormone levels regularly

Intermittent fasting in various forms appears to be healthy for women. However, serious side effects like increased appetite, mood swings, decreased concentration, and bad breath has been documented in some studies. Whether some women have confirmed a complete cessation of their menstrual cycle. As a result, it's critical that women who are experiencing a quick monitor their hormones regularly. If a woman's mood or health condition changes significantly, she should stop fasting immediately and see a doctor.

6.1.5   Need to get in the Right Mindset

Many people strive to maintain their intermittent fasting goals because they lack the required mentality. They give up before they even notice the changes they want.

Intermittent fasting, also known as IF, isn't and shouldn't be a one-time program. In reality, you must be consistent and incorporate it into your daily routine.

It would be best if you also were certain of your objectives. Do you, for example, use intermittent fasting to lose weight? These goals will help you create targets for determining whether or not

IF is effective for you. Those who adhere to intermittent fasting reap several health benefits. It's not only a perfect diet plan for losing body fat because it lets you consume fewer calories, but it could also boost your overall health. According to a report, fasting can help people with obesity lower their blood pressure.

Intermittent fasting of 3 to 24 weeks has been shown in other studies to help pre-diabetic people regulate their blood sugar, glucose, and insulin levels. Fasting has also been linked to a lower risk of type 2 diabetes, certain heart diseases, including non-alcoholic liver cancer. It can also help to maintain memory and delay the progression of Alzheimer's disease. Repeated short-term fasting has also been shown in animal research to prolong lifespan.

Some people, however, do not consider themselves as candidates. Children and people under the age of 18, pregnant mothers, breastfeeding women, people with weakened immune systems, and people with other underlying health issues are all examples.

Fasting should be avoided by someone with disordered eating or background of disordered eating, as irregular eating habits and periods of just not eating can cause a worsening of their condition. Even if you're in good health, you shouldn't start IF without first consulting your doctor. Before you start, make sure you're in good physical condition.

6.1.6 Decide how you'd like to fast

Intermittent fasting, as previously stated, is a cyclical cycle of fasting that includes calorie restriction or food abstinence, accompanied by food intake. We have various intermittent fasting plans based on this definition. Longer periods of fasting, on the other hand, may result in the development of gallstones. Women, irrespective of their weight, are at a higher risk. It's also possible that skipping breakfast isn't the best option for everybody. According to a report published by that of the European Society of Cardiology, such habit may be linked to atherosclerosis, a disease marked by artery narrowing and hardening.

If you want to miss breakfast, make sure to stay hydrated during the day and start slowly, paying attention to body language for energy crashes. If you're having trouble getting to your next meal and finding it difficult to work in the morning with no food, you might want to reconsider your fasting strategy.

6.1.7 Maintain as much of a routine as possible

Your favorite fasting method is just as important as your dedication to the schedule. You want to pick an intermittent fasting regimen that you can stick to as much as possible.

These pointers can be useful:

- Make dinner the last meal so that your fasting time is extended.

- Make a schedule for the week's events. Switch your fasting time the day before if you intend to join a birthday lunch on Friday.

- Keep yourself occupied so that you don't end up grabbing nutrition throughout the middle of your fast.

Do you want to exercise? If possible, do after the quick.

6.1.8 Maintain hydration

Hunger is one of the immediate consequences of intermittent fasting because you're more likely to jeopardize your performance when you're hungry. Drink anything in between to stop it IF it allows you to drink herbal teas, tea, and water while fasting. You can also try a drink made with alkalizing greens like wheatgrass, kale, broccoli, Spirulina, butternut squash, collard greens, green beans, beet greens, and celery which can help you refuel. You will have more energy and improved cognitive performance, better digestion, and less inflammation if you keep your body slightly alkaline.

6.1.9 Maintain Portion Control

You don't have the luxury of obesity during your non-fast time because you're on an intermittent fasting diet. This merely negates the advantages of intermittent fasting.

Portion control is still essential, but it can be difficult when your stomach is grumbling. One strategy is to space out your meals so that you don't have to consume big portions during your non-fast period.

Consider the following plan if you have an 8-hour feeding window:

- Eat the first regular meal within the first hour.
- During the second hour, eat a small snack.
- Eat your second regular meal at the third hour.
- Get another quick snack at the fifth hour.
- Eat the last usual meal at the seventh hour.

Between these meals, drink plenty of water and, if it works, have used a smaller plate with improved portion control.

6.1.10 Consume the Correct Foods

Eating the right foods goes hand in hand with portion control. When IF leaves you hungry, you can reach for microwaveable meals or the nearest burger-and-fry joint. You can also drink sweetened drinks for the flavor or because you feel you need to raise your carbohydrate intake. Both of these will not provide you with the desired intermittent fasting performance. Processed foods, especially those that are ultra-processed, can make you feel even hungrier. Worse, you're growing the chances of developing metabolic problems, such as obesity.

Here are some healthy food suggestions:

Avocados and salmon are good sources of healthy fats.

Grass-fed beef, nutritious tofu, grains, peas, and lentils are good sources of nutritious, lean protein.

Pile leafy greens on your plate.

As a snack, eat some nuts.

Consider making nutritious food substitutions.

In between fasting times, some people choose to eat a low-carb, low-calorie plan to maintain fat burning and reduce the risk of weight gain. One example is the ketogenic diet.

6.1.11 Sleep Well

Sleep deprivation can also cause you to lose or not achieve your desirable intermittent fasting performance. Sleep deprivation can cause various issues, including a loss of control over calorie consumption and weight. It can increase the development of ghrelin, a hormone that increases appetite. It can also reduce the release of leptin, a hormone that helps to control hunger. Sleep deprivation can cause you to crave more cookies or other sweets. This is because it may stimulate endocannabinoid, the same form of lipid that marijuana stimulates. A minimum of eight hours of sleep is an optimal goal to strive for. If you're having trouble sleeping, make sure you're practicing healthy sleep habits like not using devices (blue light) until bed and not drinking caffeine until 4–6 hours of going to bed.

6.2 Weight Loss tips

The following suggestions will assist you in losing weight more quickly.

6.2.1 Obtain Enough Rest

The appetite hormones leptin and ghrelin are strongly influenced by sleep. So make sure you get 6-8 hours of sleep every day to keep your appetite in check and stop overeating.

6.2.2 Strengthen the body

Intermittent fasting combined with strength and weight training can speed up weight loss and improve muscle mass.

6.2.3 Sugar consumption should be reduced

Sugars and carbohydrates play a significant role in weight gain and can reduce the benefits of intermittent fasting. As a result, sugary foods and beverages should be avoided.

6.2.4 Keep a food diary

Keeping a food log will assist you in keeping track of your calories, including weight loss, while dieting. This will assist you in regulating your eating habits and daily schedule following your needs, allowing you to optimize your gains.

6.2.5 Take a probiotic supplement

Probiotics are known to help with digestive health, gut microbiome restoration, and immune system support. So, to stay balanced during intermittent fasting, sure to bring probiotic supplements. Women of all ages may benefit from intermittent fasting. If you are a woman over 50 who wants to lose the last few stubborn pounds, try intermittent fasting.

Chapter 7: Psychological Effects of Intermittent Fasting

7.1 It has the potential to affect your mood

If you've been too hungry, and who hasn't? , you're well aware that an empty stomach can lead to irritability and rage. Spend enough time without food, thanks to intermittent fasting, and your mood will begin to change. Are you irritable? This is due to low blood sugar levels and "a spike in cortisol (the stress hormone)," which occurs when people become overly hungry. Your blood sugar falls eventually spikes when "feasting" can be particularly dangerous for people with diabetes because they can lead to a loss of blood glucose regulation and interfere with diabetes treatment and insulin requirements. (It is worth noting that low-carb diets such as the keto diet can benefit people with diabetes). Are you combative? That also appears to be right. "There seems to be a hormone named neuropeptide Y which causes people to be more aggressive when they're really hungry," Albers-Bowling says, "going back to caveman days when you just got to eat if you had been fighting or your dinner."

7.2 It may make you feel even more anxious

The higher the level of cortisol in your body, the further likely you are to be depressed. According to some research, "there is some evidence that restricting dietary activity increases a stress hormone cortisol, which can induce changes in food preferences, cravings, and mood." High cortisol levels also have been related to increased fat accumulation, so IF can work against you if you're looking to lose weight.

7.3 It can make you tired

Although a small pilot study showed which intermittent fasting could boost your night, other research suggests that it is much more likely to cause sleep problems. As per a study in the journal Science and Nature of Sleep, fasting will reduce REM sleep (the super intense healing shut-eye), leading to the body's increase in cortisol and insulin. (The good news is that you can eat your path to improve sleep). Depending on the intermittent fasting strategy you use, you can avoid eating several hours before bedtime, which is a good thing because eating right before bedtime is bad for your health, leading to weight gain, acid reflux, excessive gas, and sleeping problems. However, an empty, growling stomach will make sleeping difficult.

And, let's face it, adequate sleep is important for overall mental health: "Changes in sleep behavior, quality, and length can lead to fatigue but mostly affect your mood the next day," says a researcher. (On that note, this is how your brain feels when you do not get enough sleep).

7.4 It can make you lonely

When you're unable to feed for extended periods, it can impact food-related social situations between friends and family. According to the American Psychological Association, losing out again on friend time may lead to feelings of loneliness and social alienation, leading to depression. As per the National Eating Disorders Association, those with anorexia report having fewer mates, social interests, and social support because of their diet restrictions.

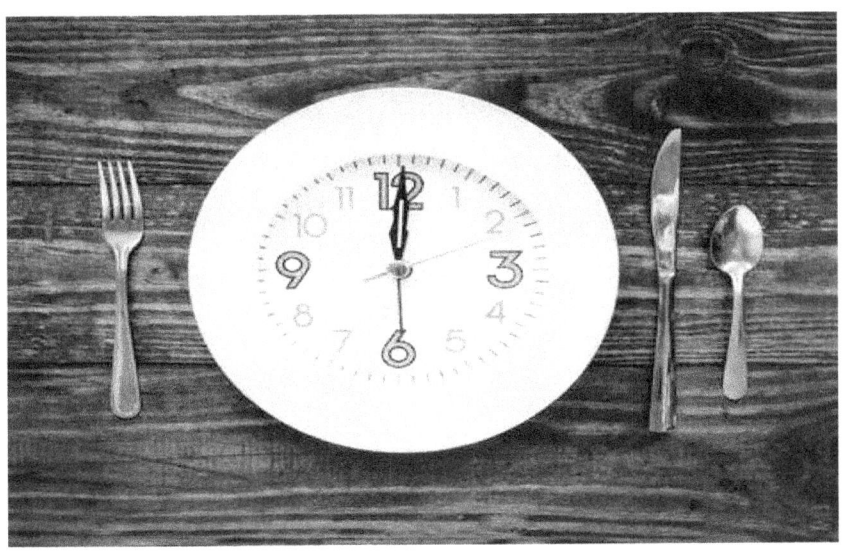

7.5 It can increase the possibility of developing eating disorders in some people.

Intermittent fasting's rigid rules about once you can and can't eat, according to the researchers, may be upsetting for someone who has had or is at risk of having an eating disorder. "At the most fundamental level, anorexia is about imposing dietary restrictions and restrictive guidelines, ignoring hunger yet fullness, and obsessing over food, all of whom can be perpetuated and compounded by Intermittent Fasting." (Also, have you ever studied orthorexia? It is an eating disorder masquerading as a balanced eating plan.) According to the researcher, the diet can also lead to "fear of losing control (with food)" or "overeating on non-restricted days." Binge eating disorder manifests itself in both of these ways. In reality, one study showed that women who reduced the caloric intake by 70% for four days but instead ate "normally" over three days had more eating-related feelings, a greater fear of losing control, and a more regular tendency for overeating throughout non-restricted hunger for just a total of four weeks. According to Albers-Bowling, Intermittent Fasting may also mask a current eating disorder. "When you say, 'Oh, I'm avoiding eating because I'm on the new fasting dieting,' people don't seem concerned. "

If you cannot take your mind off the diet or find yourself eating more than you'd if you've not fasted, intermittent fasting probably isn't for you. According to experts, intermittent fasting should be avoided entirely if you have a history of disordered eating or a poor relationship to food.

According to Hertz, intermittent fasting could be detrimental to anyone's relationship to food, but it is particularly dangerous for those with a history of disordered eating. "This is because they have a higher chance of abusing the rules and regulations to allow and exacerbate their eating disorder."

7.6 It can have an impact on your cognitive abilities

According to a study, fasting over long periods will cause you to make further rash, short-term decisions. You adjust the neurotransmitters, which are accessible throughout the brain when you fast. "As a result, restricting foods which increase serotonin levels can result in less of a feel-good chemical in your brain," which can make you more impulsive. Consider this when making food choices. In the meantime, another study of mice reported in the Published In the journal of Scientific Studies in Biosciences indicates that intermittent fasting may increase levels from certain neurotransmitters, such as serotonin, and improve learning and memory. There's contradictory evidence of the latest studies on intermittent fasting and arguments made in this paper. If you have a headache? The same. Unfortunately, there is still a ton about intermittent fasting that we do not fully comprehend.

7.7 Your perception of hunger might change

Intermittent fasting is, at its heart, about gaining mental power over hunger and, in so doing, ignoring the body's hunger signals (which, by the way, are generate by a hormone named ghrelin). According to new studies, intermittent fasting can aid with weight loss by lowering appetite and decreasing your hunger hormone ghrelin. According to animal studies, these (intermittent fasting) IF-induced increases in ghrelin can also increase dopamine levels (pleasure hormone) in the brain.

Hunger, on the other hand, is like a noisy knock on your front gate. "When you want to avoid the queues, it's as if you're covering your ears while saying, "I don't hear you; if only I wait long enough, they'll go away." Hunger appears to pound harder in the hopes of eliciting a response. If you ignore hunger signals, they will eventually stop knocking. This has a long-term negative impact on your relationship with hunger."

Chapter 8: Remedies for coping up with the drawbacks of fasting

Although the advantages of intermittent fasting greatly outweigh the disadvantages, there are a few minor aggravating adverse effects, one of which is intermittent fasting (IF) headache. You have probably had a fasting headache if you've ever been without food for an extended time (much longer than the body is used to). On your fast day or during the fasting window, headaches are more likely to occur for the following reasons:

- Hypoglycemia (Low blood sugar levels)
- Dehydration
- Electrolyte Deficiency
- Caffeine Withdrawal

On the plus side, there are many ways to handle and minimize these Disadvantages so that you do not have to avoid fasting and keep going before your goal-feeding window arrives. Below is an overview of each of these factors and treatments that have helped me and others.

The Causes will eventually fade away as you move through your fasting journey.

8.1 Hypoglycemia

When the body's sugar, glucose level falls below 70mg/dL, hypoglycemia occurs. Headaches, irritability, fatigue, dizziness, shakiness, plus hunger are all symptoms of low glucose. If you eat a high-sugar meal before the fasting window begins, you may experience a rapid rise of blood sugar followed by a rapid drop, resulting in a headache.

Remedy

Before beginning your fasting time, avoid carbs with such a high glycemic index (GI). If you want to eat high-GI carbs, eat them in the middle during your feeding window, and low-GI carbs at the end during your fasting period. Low GI carbs cause the blood sugar levels to fluctuate much less, which can help minimize the huge glucose spikes that cause intermittent fasting headaches.

8.2 Dehydration

Intermittent fasting headaches may be caused by dehydration. Water can make up 50-65 percent of the average human's body composition. This means that, in addition to oxygen, consuming water is important. Perhaps more so, the brain is composed of 75% water, and a lack of water will cause your brain to contract or shrink momentarily due to fluid loss, resulting in dehydration headaches. This pain is caused by your brain moving away from your skull, according to Medical News

Today. Headaches are one of the most common symptoms of dehydration. There are some other symptoms like:

- dark-colored urine
- reduced urination
- extreme thirst
- confusion
- dizziness
- fatigue
- dry, sticky mouth

Remedy

So, the only solution would be to drink water. You should drink at least 12 gallons of water a day, and I suggest at least one gallon if you are doing strenuous workouts.

8.3 Electrolyte Deficiency

Electrolyte imbalances are another cause of intermittent fasting headaches. Drinking electrolyte-rich water will help you stick to your quick. Electrolytes are chemical components of the body needed for various physiological functions, including muscular contractions, nerve impulses, heart function, and brain function, to name a few. Sodium, magnesium, also potassium are the three main electrolytes the body needs throughout intermittent fasting. Intermittent fasting aims to reduce insulin levels to use fat reserves for energy and lose weight. When you lower your insulin levels, your body retains less sodium and water, contributing to electrolyte imbalances. The following are some of the most common symptoms of electrolyte deficiency:

- aches and pains
- Feeling dizzy
- Confusion
- Fatigue
- Muscle spasms
- Heart pounding

This is why electrolytes must be consumed when fasting.

Remedy

We give you the general rule of thumb for eating enough sodium and keep the electrolytes balanced when fasting.

Thumb's rule:

Get at least 2000 mg of sodium per day (one to two tsp of salt). Shoot for 4000-7000 mg-s if you are physically active, either sweat a lot (2-3 tsp of salt). "Mixed with water." suggests using Himalayan salt instead of standard table salt in your water. The health benefits of Himalayan salt are well-known.

Himalayan salt and Lemon are combined in this drink to relieve headaches in minutes. This salt plus lemon drink helps to improve your immune function, boost stamina, restore alkaline balance in your body, and raise serotonin levels, in addition to resolving electrolyte imbalances.

8.4   Caffeine Withdrawal

Intermittent fasting headaches are often caused by caffeine withdrawal. When you are used to drinking multiple cups of tea and coffee every day and suddenly quit, your body may not like it, and you may experience headaches as a result.

Remedy

Caffeine is good for you! Your fast will not be broken by coffee or tea. Coffee and tea should be consumed because they help increase the pace at which we burn body fat and leave you feeling satiated. GABA (Gamma-aminobutyric acid) is a chemical found in black coffee that helps you feel healthy and relaxed. Green tea, in particular, contains a chemical named epigallocatechin - 3- gallate (EGCG), which aids in the management of your fast as well as the reduction of hunger. So, when you are hungry, grab that cup of green tea!

It is recommended that you should not use creamers or sugar in your tea or coffee. These items will break your fast, which you do not want to happen. You just do not want to consume too much caffeine. Caffeine in excess may have a harmful impact by revving up your adrenals and increasing your cortisol levels. Cortisol levels rising could lead to insulin levels rising, and intermittent fasting would aim to maintain insulin levels low so that fat stores can be activated for energy. So do not squander it by overindulging in coffee.

Chapter 9: Myths of Intermittent Fasting

9.1 Myth 1: When Intermittent Fasting, You Can't Focus

Consider the very last time we were really hungry. It wasn't likely your best zen moment.

You do not feel this "hangry" condition if you practice intermittent fasting regularly. Your hunger hormones will regulate until your cells have adapted to the use of body fat for energy. Ketones are small molecules that provide clean, usable energy to your brain as you burn body fat. It's been shown that promoting ketosis increases attention, concentration, and focus for older adults.

9.2 Myth 2: Intermittent Fasting Causes The Metabolism To Decrease

Some people believe that fasting causes the resting metabolic rate to decrease. In other words, intermittent fasting makes you burn lesser calories at rest. The fear is that you will gain weight like a three-toed sloth if you resume regular eating habits. That is what happens on calorie-restricted diets, which require you to consume 50 to 85 percent of calories your body regularly needs for a long time. Your body adjusts to the reduced energy intake and can do so for years. You have probably observed calorie restriction in effect on The Biggest Loser. While the contestants lose the weight, they almost always regain it. The show never mentions that aspect, which is inconvenient for viewers.

Is intermittent fasting the same as regular fasting? It does not seem to be the case. Non-obese people who observed alternate-day fasting retained a regular metabolic rate again for the majority of three weeks, even while burning more fat, according to a 2005 report study in the American Journal for Clinical Nutrition.

9.3 Myth 3: Everyone Can use it

Intermittent fasting is all the rage these days. In certain cases, it is sold as being helpful to all, all of the time. While fasting is generally healthy and safe for the majority of people, some groups should avoid it. The following are some of these groups: kids, pregnant and nursing women, and underweight people. The groups as mentioned above need more food, not lesser. Fasting's possible advantages are outweighed by the chance of nutrient deficiency. Those with high blood sugar must exercise caution as well. Fasting may be beneficial for this population, but medical supervision is needed to avoid extremely low blood sugar (hypoglycemia).

9.4 Myth 4: When Intermittent Fasting, You should Not Drink Water

Some religious fasts, such as Ramadan fasting, limit both food and water. Unrelated to this, various reports have emerged claiming that no-water fasts were beneficial to one's wellbeing. Due to the diuretic effect of fasting, restricting water may lead to disastrous dehydration. That's why, when supervising patients on therapeutic fasts, doctors pay careful attention to fluid intake. Electrolytes, including sodium and potassium, which are energetically ripped out during fasting, are often monitored by doctors. What's the takeaway? During a fast, drink plenty of water and take potassium and sodium supplements if the fast lasts longer than 13 or 15 hours.

9.5 Myth 5: No matter what, you'll lose weight

Contrary to common belief, intermittent fasting, even fasting in particular, does not necessarily result in weight loss. This type of mindset is a common misconception whenever it comes to these types of dieting. No know how old you've been fasting, the chances of surviving are slim to nil if you're breaking this with fries, burgers, and candy. Each fasting day should never be deemed a cheat day in order and for the diet to function.

Myth 6: When you break your fast, you can consume as much as you'd like.

Intermittent fasting, as with every other diet, is just starting a healthier way of life. Unfortunately, many people believe that they can resume their usual eating habits once their fast is over. This is in direct opposition to all of them working hard. The most interesting thing to remember when it applies to I.F. is to skip breakfast when you've broken the fast. You would have lost your fasting time if you fasted all day before dinner and only ate dinner the size of breakfast/lunch/dinner.

9.6 Myth 6: Intermittent Fasting will make you incredibly safe and fit

When combined with good practice and exercise, intermittent fasting will lead to weight loss. However, anyone adopting the diet should be mindful that it is not a successful way of losing weight independently. There is no one-size-fits-all solution. Don't take health and happiness for granted; they're things you'd work hard to keep in your life. Fasting won't give you the ideal body overnight, and even if you lose the weight, you'll have had to keep it off with healthy habits like eating better and exercising regularly.

Myth 8: Intermittent Fasting will make you incredibly safe and fit.

In long-term clinical trials, participants in the fasting groups showed no signs of hunger or dietary deficiency. The performance of the diets should be prioritized when breaking the fast. Finally, since chubby vitamins become readily accessible when absorbed through circulation from fat stores, nutritional shortages can be avoided by restricting refined, nutrient-poor diets and growing nutrient-dense, unprocessed foods.

9.7 Myth 7: Intermittent Fasting is nothing more than starvation

Fasting is a conscious act in which one refrains from feeding for a specified period. True starvation happens when food is unavailable for an unknown period, and the person has little control over the situation. When people fast, their endogenous insulin levels decrease, meaning that they are not hungry and get a regular calorie through fat stores.

9.8 Myth 8: The most significant food of the day will be breakfast

Breakfast is needed to give you the extra boost you need to get your day started. If you don't eat first thing every morning, your body will respond by raising adrenaline (growth hormone) but cortisol levels, causing the liver to produce glucose, giving you the energy those who need to get through the day. As a consequence, breakfast isn't as important as it once was. Breakfast is typically associated with eating first thing in the morning. It is much more socially acceptable to acknowledge that if one breaks the overnight soon, it's doesn't matter whenever the phrase is decomposed (breakfast).

9.9 Myth 9: Intermittent Fasting Causes Overreacting

You'll be hungry after a short. Many people believe that this hunger would lead to overeating. The proof, on the other hand, refutes this concern. Ad libitum feeding refers to the process of allowing participants to consume as much as they want during a fasting study. They eat to their hearts' content and still lose weight. Many intermittent fasting protocols would cause you to eat less rather than more. As a result of the moderate calorie restriction, you'll lose weight gradually without slowing down your metabolism.

9.10 Myth 10: If You Fast, You Will Not Gain Muscle

Fasting does not seem to be the only way to gain muscle mass. Do you still need to pounds protein shakes? Protein is necessary, but it is not needed all of the time. In one 2019 report, for example, healthy women who fasted 16/8 gained the same amount of strength and muscle as women who ate on a more traditional schedule. Here's the deal: In times of shortage, the body works overtime to conserve muscle. When you fast, your body fat (rather than muscle) is used to meet your energy needs.

Consider this: if we burned across muscle throughout a fast, our forefathers would have been unable to hunt!

9.11 Myth 11: Lack Of Energy Is Caused By intermittent fasting

Food is a source of energy. Would your energy levels fall if you don't have them?

Yes, eventually. When the fast intermittently, though, your cells switch to a different source of energy: body fat. There's plenty of it to go around. That's right. Even a thin person (e.g., 150 pounds of 10% body fat) has significant fat reserves to meet energy demands when fasting. Fifteen pounds of fat equals over 60,000 calories for energy if you do the math! In reality, many people claim that exercising while fasted gives them more energy. After a big meal, blood is redirected away from muscles and into digestive organs, making sense.

Conclusion

In conclusion, intermittent fasting will do more benefit to your body than any other diet. It will boost your metabolism, help you save time and improve your cognition too. It has also been proven to reverse the sign of aging, making you feel and look a lot younger. You can follow so many different methods and start your transformation regardless of the type of fasting you chose. Being well while you do eat is important. During fasting cycles, all of the approaches we've discussed allow you to eat little, making it much more necessary to keep hydrated. Coffee and water are mostly acceptable beverages; however, they eliminate high in carbs. If you are still adding food high in sugar and calories, it will do no good. Choosing to stay hydrated when fasting ensures you get the most from intermittent fasting.

This book will help you choose the best method for you and help you restrict the number of calories, but it's best to start slow as you're in your 50s, and we don't want you to put your body into a lot of stress. If your body fasting is a new concept, it will always take time to get used to it. It will be best to consult your doctor before starting intermittent fasting.

www.ingramcontent.com/pod-product-compliance
Lightning Source LLC
Chambersburg PA
CBHW070805220526
45466CB00002B/557